T0191987

Neuro-Oncology Explained Through Multiple Choice Questions

Your bonus with the purchase of this book

With the purchase of this book, you can use our "SN Flashcards" app to access questions free of charge in order to test your learning and check your understanding of the contents of the book.
To use the app, please follow the instructions below:

1. Go to **https://flashcards.springernature.com/login**
2. Create an user account by entering your e-mail adress and assiging a password.
3. Use the link provided in one of the first chapters to access your SN Flashcards set.

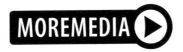

Your personal SN Flashcards link is provided in one of the first chapters.

If the link is missing or does not work, please send an e-mail with the subject "**SN Flashcards**" and the book title to **customerservice@springernature.com**.

Joe M Das

Neuro-Oncology Explained Through Multiple Choice Questions

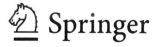 Springer

Joe M Das
Consultant Neurosurgeon
Bahrain Specialist Hospital
Juffair, Bahrain

ISBN 978-3-031-13255-1   ISBN 978-3-031-13253-7   (eBook)
https://doi.org/10.1007/978-3-031-13253-7

This Springer imprint is published by the registered company Springer Nature Switzerland AG
The registered company address is: Gewerbestrasse 11, 6330 Cham, Switzerland

Dedicated to my late father,
Dr Mariadas S.

Foreword

The rapid progress of neuro-oncology and the numerous researches conducted in this field make it next to impossible for a neurosurgeon or an oncologist to remain up to date.

I have known the main author, Joe M. Das, since the time he had been doing a post-doctoral fellowship in skull base neurosurgery at the Sree Chitra Tirunal Institute for Medical Sciences and Technology. It is indeed a pleasure and an honor for me to be invited to write a foreword to this excellent book, *Neuro-oncology Explained Through Multiple Choice Questions*.

This book is highly scientific, educational, and informative. Almost all the topics in the field have been included, and the multiple-choice question (MCQ) format makes it more appealing for the reader to test their knowledge.

For a question author, a well-crafted MCQ is not always just about writing the best correct answer, it is also about creating deeply convincing false answers or distractors. This takes more time than a simple fill-in-the-blank or essay question. I highly appreciate the effort put forth by Dr Das and his co-authors in completing such amazing work with precise and updated explanations.

As a professor in neurosurgery, I came to know many finer details in neuro-oncology after going through the book. It delivers comprehensive information on neuro-oncology in the form of brainstorming questions, succinct explanations, and answers.

I am sure it will be wonderful teaching and learning material for everyone working in the fields of neuroscience and oncology—residents, trainees, faculty, and consultants.

I heartily congratulate Dr Das for this outstanding work and hope he keeps it up with newer editions and contributes to the growth and development of neuro-oncology. I wish him all the best.

Suresh Nair
Former Dean & Prof (Senior Grade) of Neurosurgery
Sree Chitra Tirunal Institute of Medical Sciences
Trivandrum, India

Hinduja National Hospital
Mumbai, Maharashtra, India

Preface

This is our humble attempt to summarize the major neurosurgical concepts in neuro-oncology with the help of multiple-choice questions. I sincerely thank all the contributors who have given their best in adding quality content. We have tried to keep the facts as simple as possible, especially the molecular classification. Medical science, especially neuro-oncology, is a rapidly changing field. We have taken efforts to keep the contents up to date. One peculiarity of the book is that we have introduced many updates and nuances, which may be difficult to comprehend.

Hot topics like artificial intelligence and nanotheranostics are added.

This book is intended for those in neurosurgery and oncology training and will act as a refresher for consultant neurosurgeons, neurologists, and medical/radiation oncologists. The book is written assuming that the reader already knows the basics of neurosurgery and neuro-oncology. We are sure that this book will help to increase your existing level of knowledge on the subject and inspire reading.

It is almost impossible to include every topic in neuro-oncology in a single book. This book excludes spinal and pediatric oncology.

The book contains both multiple-choice and matching questions, both formats are likely to be interesting to the reader. We have tried to avoid giving the names of trials, and percentages have been rounded off.

In addition, we would invite readers to explore the Springer Nature Flashcards available with individual chapters. The cards are intended to help with consolidating knowledge from the text. Download the Springer Nature Flashcards app for free (https://flashcards.springernature.com/login) and use this exclusive additional material to consolidate your knowledge.

"*Errare humanum est.*"—Latin proverb.

As mentioned by Dade Lunsford, the field of neurosurgery has been part of an enormous paradigm shift over the last decade of the twentieth century and the initial years of the twenty-first century. We have started applying molecular and laboratory data in the operating room rather than going back to the laboratory from the operating room. We totally stand by his concept and have included more molecular aspects of oncology in our book.

We sincerely wish you happy reading.

Juffair, Bahrain

Joe M. Das

Acknowledgment

I would like to thank my wife (Dr Salini) and daughter (Miss Aarika) for always being there for me and excusing me for doing academic activities during times that could have been spent with them.

I thank my mother (Ms Daisy) and my friends (Drs Prasanth TS, Kiran N and Sreeganesh K) for supporting me in all the things I do.

Abbreviations

^{18}F-FDG	2-Deoxy-2-[fluorine-18]fluoro-D-glucose
^{18}F-FDOPA	3,4-Dihydroxy-6-(18F) fluoro-L-phenylalanine
3D	Three dimensional
ABC	ATP-binding cassette
ABR	Auditory brainstem response
ACTH	Adrenocorticotropic hormone
ACVR1	Activin A receptor Type 1
ADC	Apparent diffusion coefficient
AED	Antiepileptic drug
AFP	Alpha-fetoprotein
AIDS	Acquired immunodeficiency syndrome
ALKBH5	alkB homolog 5 (alkB - Alkane hydroxylase gene)
APC	Adenomatous polyposis coli
ASV	Anterior septal vein
ATM	Ataxia telangiectasia mutated
ATP	Adenosine triphosphate
ATRX	Alpha-thalassemia/mental retardation, X-linked
BAER	Brainstem auditory evoked response
BAP1	BRCA1-associated protein 1 (BRCA1 - Breast cancer type 1)
BCOR	BCL6 Corepressor (Bcl-6 - B-cell lymphoma 6)
b-FGF	Basic fibroblast growth factor
BMI	Body Mass Index
BMP	Bone morphogenetic protein
B-RAF	Rapidly accelerated fibrosarcoma-B
BRG-1	Brahma-related gene-1
BTK	Bruton tyrosine kinase
BTSC	Brain tumor stem cell
C11orf95 (ZFTA)	Zinc finger translocation associated
CARD11	Caspase recruitment domain family member 11
CD	Cluster of differentiation
Cdk	Cyclin-dependent kinase

CDKN2A	Cyclin-dependent kinase inhibitor 2A
CIC	Capicua transcriptional repressor
CITED2	Cbp/P300 interacting transactivator with Glu/Asp rich carboxy-terminal domain 2
CMAP	Compound muscle action potentials
CNS	Central nervous system
CP	Carotid paraganglioma
CP	Cerebellopontine
CREB	cAMP-response element-binding protein (cAMP—Cyclic adenosine monophosphate)
CREBBP	Cyclic adenosine monophosphate response element binding protein binding protein
CRL4^{CRBN}	Cullin-Ring ligase 4 E3 ubiquitin ligase complex
CSF	Cerebrospinal fluid
CT	Computed tomogram
CTLA4	Cytotoxic T-lymphocyte-associated protein 4
CTNNB1	Catenin beta 1
CXCL12	C-X-C motif chemokine 12
CXCR-4	C-X-C chemokine receptor type 4
DAL-1	Differentially expressed in adenocarcinoma of the lung-1
DCC	Deleted in colorectal carcinoma
DGCR8	DiGeorge syndrome critical region 8
DICER	Gene encoding endoribonuclease dicer
DLK1	Delta-like non-canonical notch ligand 1
DNA	Deoxyribonucleic acid
DROSHA	Gene encoding drosha ribonuclease III
DTI	Diffusion tensor imaging
E.coli	*Escherichia coli*
ECM	Extracellular matrix
ECOG	Eastern Cooperative Oncology Group
EGFR	Epidermal growth factor receptor
EMA	Epithelial membrane antigen
EORTC	The European Organisation for Research and Treatment of Cancer
ERCC2	Excision repair cross-complementation group 2
ERK	Extracellular signal-regulated kinases
ETV	Endoscopic third ventriculostomy
EZHIP	Enhancer of zest homologs inhibitory protein
FET	FUS (Fused in liposarcoma), EWS (Ewing sarcoma) and TAF15 (TATA binding-associated factor 15)
FGFR	Fibroblast growth factor receptor
FIPA	Familial isolated pituitary adenoma
FLAIR	Fluid-attenuated inversion recovery
fMRI	Functional magnetic resonance imaging

FOS	FBJ Murine osteosarcoma viral oncogene homolog (FBJ - Finkel-Biskis-Jinkins)
FOXR2	Forkhead box R2
FTO	Fat mass and obesity associated
GAP	GTPase-accelerating protein
GBM	Glioblastoma
Gd	Gadolinium
GDP	Guanosine diphosphate
GFAP	Glial fibrillary acidic protein
GFI1	Growth factor independence-1
GH	Growth hormone
GI	Gastrointestinal
GLI	Glioma-associated oncogene
GLK1	Glucokinase-1
GNA11	G protein subunit alpha 11
GNAQ	Guanine nucleotide-binding protein alpha-Q
GNAT1	G Protein subunit alpha transducin 1
GRE	Gradient echo sequence
GTP	Guanosine triphosphate
Gy	Gray
H3 G34	Codon 34 in the H3 histone, family 3A
H3K27M	Lys-27-Met mutations in histone 3 genes
HER2	Human epidermal growth factor receptor 2
HGF-SF	Hepatocyte growth factor (HGF) or scatter factor (SF)
HGG	High-grade glioma
HHT	Hereditary hemorrhagic telangiectasia
HIF	Hypoxia-inducible factor
HIV	Human immunodeficiency virus
HMGB1	High mobility group protein B1
HNP	Head-and-neck paragangliomas
hnRNPC	Heterogeneous nuclear ribonucleoprotein C
HSP	Heat shock protein
HSV	Herpes simplex virus
ICG	Indocyanine green
ICV	Internal cerebral vein
IDH	Isocitrate dehydrogenase
IFN	Interferon
IHC	Immunohistochemistry
IL	Interleukin
INI1	Integrase interactor 1
IR	Infrared
ISF	Interstitial fluid
JC virus	John Cunningham virus
JP	Jugular paraganglioma
KBTBD4	Kelch repeat and BTB domain-containing 4

KIAA	Kazusa DNA Research Institute
KLF4	Krüppel-like factor 4
L1CAM	L1 Cell adhesion molecule
LAM	Lymphangioleiomyomatosis
LDH	Lactate dehydrogenase
LGG	Low grade glioma
LP	Laryngeal paraganglioma
mAb	Monoclonal antibody
MAPK	Mitogen-activated protein kinase
MBEN	Medulloblastoma with extensive nodularity
MEK	Mitogen-activated protein kinase kinase
MEN1	Multiple endocrine neoplasia 1
MET	Mesenchymal epithelial transition factor
METTL3	Methyltransferase-like 3
MGMT	O-6-Methylguanine-DNA methyltransferase
MIB1	Mindbomb homolog 1
miRNA	microRNA
MLF	Medial longitudinal fasciculus
MLH1	mutL homolog 1
MMP	Matrix metalloproteinase
MNX1	Motor neuron and pancreas homeobox 1
MRA	Magnetic Resonance Angiogram
MRI	Magnetic resonance imaging
mRNA	Messenger RNA
MSH2	MutS homolog 2
MTD	Mean tumor diameter
mTOR	Mechanistic target of rapamycin
MYB	Myeloblastosis
MYBL1	MYB proto-oncogene Like 1
MYCN	Master regulator of cell cycle entry and proliferative metabolism-N
MYD88	Myeloid differentiation primary response 88
NAA	N-acetylaspartate
NAB2	NGFI-A binding protein 2 (NGF – Nerve growth factor)
NADPH	Nicotinamide adenine dinucleotide phosphate
NANOG	Tìr nan Òg (the mythical Celtic land of youth)
NBS	Nijmegen breakage syndrome
NCAM	Neural cell adhesion molecule
NE	Neutrophil elastase
NEO1	Neogenin 1
NeuN	Neuronal nuclei
NF1	Neurofibromatosis type 1
NIH	National Institutes of Health
NIR	Near-Infrared
NLGN	Neuroligin

NRAS	Rat sarcoma virus-N
NSAID	Nonsteroidal anti-inflammatory drugs
OC	*Ordospora colligata*
OLIG2	Oligodendrocyte transcription factor 2
OPG	Optic pathway glioma
PAK	p21-Activated serine/threonine kinases
PAS	Periodic acid-Schiff
PCNSL	Primary central nervous system lymphoma
PDGFRA	Platelet-derived growth factor receptor alpha
PET	Positron Emission Tomogram
PI3K	Phosphoinositide 3-kinase
PIK3CA	Phosphatidylinositol-4,5-bisphosphate 3-kinase, catalytic subunit alpha
PIT-1	Pituitary-specific positive transcription factor 1
PMS2	Postmeiotic segregation increased 2
PNET	Primitive neuroectodermal tumor
PPT	Pineal parenchymal tumor
PRAME	Preferentially expressed antigen of melanoma
PRKAR1A	Protein kinase CAMP-dependent type I regulatory subunit alpha
PRKCA	Protein kinase C alpha
PTCH1	Protein patched homolog 1
PTEN	Phosphatase and tensin homolog
PTPR	Papillary tumor of the pineal region
PUMA	Programmable Universal Machine for Assembly
PVS-RIPO	Poliovirus Sabin rhinovirus IRES poliovirus open reading frame (IRES - Internal ribosomal entry site)
QD	Quantum Dot
RB1	Retinoblastoma 1
RBM15	RNA-binding motif protein 15
RCT	Randomized controlled trial
RELA	v-rel avian reticuloendotheliosis viral oncogene homolog A
RNA	Ribonucleic acid
ROSA	Robotic surgical assistant
rRNA	Ribosomal ribonucleic acid
SDF-1	Stromal cell-derived factor 1
SDH	Succinate dehydrogenase
SEGA	Subependymal giant cell astrocytoma
SF-1	Steroidogenic factor 1
SHH	Sonic hedgehog signaling molecule
SIADH	Syndrome of inappropriate ADH secretion (ADH - Antidiuretic hormone)
SLC12A1	Solute carrier family 12 member 1
SMA	Supplementary motor area

SMARCA4	SWI/SNF-related, matrix-associated, actin-dependent regulator of chromatin, subfamily A, member 4
SMARCB1	SWI/SNF-related, matrix associated, actin-dependent regulator of chromatin, subfamily B, member 1 (SWI/SNF - SWItch/Sucrose non-fermentable)
SMARCE1	SWI/SNF-related, matrix-associated, actin-dependent regulator of chromatin, subfamily E, member 1
SNP	Single nucleotide polymorphism
snRNA	Small nuclear RNA
SOX-2	Sex determining region Y-box 2
SRS	Stereotactic radiosurgery
STAT	Signal transducer and activator of transcription
SUFU	Suppressor of fused
SWI	Susceptibility-weighted imaging
SWS	Sturge-Weber syndrome
TERT	Telomerase reverse transcriptase
TGF	Transforming growth factor
TIFF-1	Trefoil factor 1
TIMP-1	Tissue inhibitor of metalloproteinases 1
TMZ	Temozolomide
TOX	Thymocyte selection-associated high mobility group box
TP	Tympanic paraganglioma
TP53	Tumor protein P53
T-PIT	Pituitary-restricted transcription factor
TRAF7	TNF receptor-associated factor 7 (TNF - tumor necrosis factor)
TSC	Tuberous sclerosis
TSH	Thyroid-stimulating hormone
TTF-1	Thyroid transcription factor-1
UBO	Unidentified bright object
UCLA	The University of California at Los Angeles
UNC	Uncoordinated
US FDA	The United States Food and Drug Administration
USP8	Ubiquitin-specific peptidase 8
VEGF	Vascular endothelial growth factor
VHL	Von Hippel-Lindau
VIRMA	Vir-like M6A methyltransferase associated
VP	Vagal paraganglioma
VTE	Venous thromboembolism
WHO	World Health Organization
WNT	Wingless-related integration site—wg (from the Drosophila gene wingless) and int (from the proto-oncogene integration-1)
WTAP	Wilm tumor 1 (WT1)-associating protein
XRT	Radiotherapy
YAP1	Yes-associated protein 1

YTHDC2	YTH domain containing 2
YTHDF2	YTH N6-Methyladenosine RNA binding protein 2 (YTH - YT521-B homology)
ZC3H13	Zinc finger CCCH-type containing 13
α KG	α-Ketoglutarate
β-hCG	Beta human chorionic gonadotropin

Contents

Contributors

Ebtesam Abdulla Department of Neurosurgery, Salmaniya Medical Complex, Manama, Bahrain

Amit Agrawal Department of Neurosurgery, All India Institute of Medical Sciences, Bhopal, Madhya Pradesh, India

Abduelmenem Alashkham Edinburgh Medical School, The University of Edinburgh, Edinburgh, UK

Jacek Baj Chair and Department of Anatomy, Medical University of Lublin, Lublin, Poland

Joe M. Das Consultant Neurosurgeon, Bahrain Specialist Hospital, Juffair, Bahrain

Dia R. Halalmeh Department of Neurosurgery, Hurley Medical Center, Flint, MI, USA

Ryan M. Hess Department of Neurosurgery, Jacobs School of Medicine and Biomedical Sciences, University at Buffalo, Buffalo, NY, USA

Department of Neurosurgery, Buffalo General Medical Center, Kaleida Health, Buffalo, NY, USA

Mohammed Jawhari Neurosurgery Resident, King Fahad General Hospital, Medina, Saudi Arabia

Amr Maani Department of Anatomy, Medical University of Lublin, Lublin, Poland

Marc D. Moisi Department of Neurosurgery, Hurley Medical Center, Flint, MI, USA

Luis Rafael Moscote-Salazar Colombian Clinical Research Group in Neurocritical Care, Bogota, Colombia

Ahmed A. Najjar College of Medicine, Taibah University, Medina, Saudi Arabia

Rajesh Krishna Pathiyil Department of Clinical Neurosciences, University of Calgary, Calgary, AB, Canada

Daulat Singh Department of Radiation Oncology, Govt Doon Medical College & Hospital, Dehradun, Uttarakhand, India

Mohamed A. R. Soliman Department of Neurosurgery, Faculty of Medicine, Cairo University, Cairo, Egypt

Chapter 1
Classification of Brain Tumors

Joe M Das

1. Which of the following is not a characteristic feature of a diffuse midline glioma?

   (a) Has a glial phenotype
   (b) More common in children
   (c) H3K27M mutation is seen
   (d) IDH2 mutation is seen

   Answer: d

   Diffuse midline glioma, H3 K27-altered is a new entity added in 2016 and modified in the 2021 WHO classification.

   The Criteria for Diagnosis are

   - K27M mutation in either the H3 Histone Family Member 3A (H3F3A) or Histone Cluster 1 H3 Family Member B/C (HIST1H3B/C) gene
   - Have a glial phenotype
   - Be located in the midline and
   - Show a diffuse growth/infiltrating pattern

   Other points about H3 K27M mutations and diffuse midline gliomas:

   - Not exclusive to midline gliomas
   - Occur primarily in children
   - Prognosis is very poor
   - 2-year survival rate is below 10%
   - Mean survival of 9 months
   - Other changes (TP53, ACVR1, PDGFRA, EGFR, EZHIP mutations) can also define this tumor entity in addition to the K27M mutations.

J. M. Das (✉)
Consultant Neurosurgeon, Bahrain Specialist Hospital, Juffair, Bahrain
e-mail: neurosurgeon@doctors.org.uk

© The Author(s), under exclusive license to Springer Nature Switzerland AG 2023
J. M. Das, *Neuro-Oncology Explained Through Multiple Choice Questions*,
https://doi.org/10.1007/978-3-031-13253-7_1

According to the latest WHO classification, pediatric-type diffuse gliomas have been classified into low-grade and high-grade:

Pediatric-type diffuse low-grade gliomas	Pediatric-type diffuse high-grade gliomas
• Diffuse astrocytoma, MYB- or MYBL1-altered	• Diffuse midline glioma, H3 K27-altered
• Angiocentric glioma	• Diffuse hemispheric glioma, H3 G34-mutant
• Polymorphous low-grade neuroepithelial tumor of the young (PLNTY)	• Diffuse pediatric-type high-grade glioma, H3-wildtype and IDH-wildtype
• Diffuse low-grade glioma, MAPK pathway-altered	• Infant-type hemispheric glioma

The term "glioblastoma" is no longer used in the pediatric setting.

2. Which of the following is false with regard to IDH mutation?

   (a) Glioblastomas with IDH1/IDH2 mutations are termed primary glioblastomas
   (b) The overall survival of IDH wild-type grade 3 astrocytoma is worse than IDH mutant grade 4 tumor
   (c) Almost 90% of the IDH mutations involve IDH1R132H
   (d) IDH1/IDH2 mutations occur at a lower frequency in glioblastoma multiforme when compared to grade 2 and 3 astrocytomas

   Answer: a

   Adult-type diffuse gliomas are classified as follows in 2021 WHO classification:

• Astrocytoma, IDH-mutant—graded as WHO grades 2, 3, or 4 (the presence of CDKN2A/B homozygous deletion results in a CNS WHO grade of 4)
• Oligodendroglioma, IDH-mutant, and 1p/19q-codeleted
• Glioblastoma, IDH-wildtype

   IDH1 gene—located on 2q34 (cytosol); IDH2 gene—located on 15q26.1 (mitochondria) converts isocitrate to α-ketoglutarate, producing NADPH (outside the normal citric acid cycle). → α-KG needed for prolyl hydroxylases to hydroxylate and promote the degradation of Hypoxia-inducible factor (HIF)-1 α.

   • Gain-of-function mutation of IDH1 → Isocitrate to D-2-hydroxyglutarate (abnormal) → Inhibits histone demethylation and affects the level of HIF-1 α → Impaired cellular differentiation.
   • Glioma precursor cell

      → IDH1 mutation +1p19q deletion → Grade 2 oligodendroglioma
      → IDH1 and p53 mutation → Grade 2 astrocytoma → Secondary GBM
      → EGFR amplification, PTEN deletion → Primary GBM

- Gliomas with mutated IDH1 and IDH2 have improved prognoses compared to gliomas with wild-type IDH.
- IDH1/IDH2 mutations are less common in glioblastomas compared to grade 2 and 3 diffuse astrocytomas, oligodendrogliomas, and oligoastrocytomas.
- The most common form of IDH mutation is a missense one in IDH1 (Arginine at position 132 → Histidine) (IDH1 R132H). This accounts for 90% of the IDH mutations in gliomas and is being used for immunohistochemical staining.
- IDH-mutated glioma shows markedly reduced glycolysis—the metabolic hallmark of highly proliferating malignancies.
- Outside the central nervous system, IDH mutations are found in acute myeloid leukemia, intrahepatic cholangiocarcinoma, and central/periosteal chondrosarcoma.

3. A patient undergoes resection of a frontal lesion. The preoperative diagnosis was oligodendroglioma. On histological examination, the lesion appears to be a low-grade astrocytoma. Which of the following feature if present, would suggest a grade 4 behavior with a poor prognosis of this tumor?

(a) The presence of TERT promoter mutation
(b) EGFR gene amplification
(c) Combined gain of whole chromosome 7 and loss of chromosome 10
(d) All the above

Answer: d

The Gliomas, Glioneuronal Tumors, and Neuronal Tumors are Divided into Six Different Families in the 2021 WHO Classification

• Adult-type diffuse gliomas
• Pediatric-type diffuse low-grade gliomas
• Pediatric-type diffuse high-grade gliomas
• Circumscribed astrocytic gliomas
• Glioneuronal and neuronal tumors; and
• Ependymomas

The following factors in a histologically lower grade, diffuse, IDH-wildtype astrocytoma make it behave like a WHO grade 4 glioblastoma

- The presence of a TERT promoter mutation and/or
- EGFR gene amplification and/or
- Combined gain of whole chromosome 7 plus loss of whole chromosome 10

Points to remember on TERT, ATRX, and TP53:

- Oligodendrogliomas (IDH-mutant, 1p/19q-codeleted) have activating mutations in the telomerase reverse transcriptase gene (TERT) promoter region.
- Astrocytomas (IDH-mutant) frequently carry an alpha-thalassemia/mental retardation syndrome X-linked gene (ATRX—negative staining by IHC) and a tumor protein p53 gene (TP53—positive staining by IHC) mutation.

4. Which of the following mutations is found in the majority of pediatric supratentorial ependymomas?

   (a) EGFR
   (b) ATRX
   (c) TERT
   (d) ZFTA

   Answer: d

   There are seven subgroups of ependymal tumors, based on DNA methylation profiling analysis:

   Supratentorial ependymoma
   Supratentorial ependymoma, ZFTA fusion-positive
   Supratentorial ependymoma, YAP1 fusion-positive
   Posterior fossa ependymoma
   Posterior fossa ependymoma, group PFA
   Posterior fossa ependymoma, group PFB
   Spinal ependymoma
   Spinal ependymoma, MYCN-amplified
   Myxopapillary ependymoma
   Subependymoma (encompassing spinal, supratentorial, and infratentorial).

   Supratentorial ependymoma, ZFTA fusion-positive:

   - Majority of pediatric supratentorial ependymal tumors
   - Fusion of RELA + effector of NF-jB signaling + C11orf95 → activation of NF kappa B pathway
   - Fusion secondary to chromothripsis (massive and clustered genomic rearrangements) of chromosome 11
   - L1CAM and cyclin D1 expression are useful surrogate markers.
   - Has a predilection for lateral and third ventricles and is associated with a worse outcome

   Points to remember on ependymomas:

   - The most common genomic aberration in pediatric intracranial ependymomas is the gain of chromosome 1q.
   - The likely cells of origin for ependymoma are the Radial Glial Cells.
   - The term "anaplastic ependymoma" is no longer used.
   - The myxopapillary ependymoma is now considered CNS WHO grade 2.

5. Match the following mutations with their corresponding frequently associated tumor

| (a) BRAF V600E | Aggressive meningiomas |
| (b) CTNNB1 | Atypical teratoid/rhabdoid tumor |

(c) MYB	Diffuse meningeal melanocytic tumors
(d) PRKCA	Pilocytic astrocytoma
(e) NAB2-STAT6 gene fusion	Diffuse meningeal melanocytic tumors
(f) TERT promoter mutation	Chordoid glioma
(g) NRAS	Solitary fibrous tumor and hemangiopericytoma
(h) FGFR1	Angiocentric glioma
(i) SMARCB1/SMARCA4 loss	Adamantinomatous craniopharyngioma
(j) KIAA1549-BRAF gene fusion	Papillary craniopharyngioma

Answer:

(a) BRAF V600E	Papillary craniopharyngioma
(b) CTNNB1	Adamantinomatous craniopharyngioma
(c) MYB	Angiocentric glioma
(d) PRKCA	Chordoid glioma
(e) NAB2-STAT6 gene fusion	Solitary fibrous tumor and hemangiopericytoma
(f) TERT promoter mutation	Aggressive meningiomas
(g) NRAS	Diffuse meningeal melanocytic tumors
(h) FGFR1	Dysembryoplastic neuroepithelial tumor
(i) SMARCB1/SMARCA4 loss	Atypical teratoid/rhabdoid tumor
(j) KIAA1549-BRAF gene fusion	Pilocytic astrocytoma

6. Which of the following is true regarding TERT mutation?

   (a) Present in almost all IDH-mutant, 1p/19q-codeleted oligodendrogliomas
   (b) Frequent in IDH-wildtype GBM
   (c) TERT promoter mutation in histologically lower-grade, IDH-wildtype astrocytoma indicates aggressive behavior ('molecular glioblastoma')
   (d) All the above

   Answer: d

   TERT (Telomerase Reverse Transcriptase) (5p15.33):

   - The most frequently mutated gene in gliomas (oligodendrogliomas and primary GBM).
   - *TERT*p mutations are mostly associated with poor outcomes, except for 1p19q codeleted grade 2 and grade 3, and *EGFR* amplified grade 3 and grade 4.
   - Found mostly in glioblastomas (IDH wildtype, 1p19q not co-deleted) and oligodendrogliomas (IDH mutant, 1p19q co-deleted)
   - If a tumor is IDH mutated, the key differentiating factor that delineates an oligodendroglioma from an astrocytoma is 1p/19q codeletion.
   - Triple positive low-grade glioma (positive for TERT, IDH, and 1p/19q co-deletion) have the best overall survival. LGG with TERT mutation alone has the worst survival.

7. Which of the following is the correct order of chance of survival of different grades of astrocytomas?

    (a) IDH-wild grade 3 > IDH-mutant grade 3 > IDH-wild grade 4 > IDH-mutant grade 4
    (b) IDH-mutant grade 3 > IDH-wild grade 3 > IDH-mutant grade 4 > IDH-wild grade 4
    (c) IDH-mutant grade 3 > IDH-mutant grade 4 > IDH-wild grade 3 > IDH-wild grade 4
    (d) IDH-wild grade 3 > IDH-wild grade 4 > IDH-mutant grade 3 > IDH-mutant grade 4

    Answer: c

    Grade 2 IDH mutant and 1p19q co-deleted have the best prognosis.

8. Which of the following histological types is not included in IDH-wild type glioblastoma?

    (a) Gliomatosis cerebri
    (b) Epithelioid glioblastoma
    (c) Giant cell glioblastoma
    (d) Gliosarcoma

    Answer: a

    The three recognized variants of glioblastoma are:

    - Giant cell glioblastoma
    - Gliosarcoma
    - Epithelioid glioblastoma

    The term "gliomatosis cerebri" has been removed from the latest WHO (2016) classification.

    Epithelioid glioblastoma:

    - New addition to the WHO 2016 and recognized in the current classification.
    - Occurs in younger patients
    - Half of them show BRAF V600E mutations
    - Differential diagnoses are anaplastic pleomorphic xanthoastrocytomas, rhabdoid meningiomas, atypical teratoid/rhabdoid tumors, metastatic tumors, and melanomas.

9. Which gene mutation is not included in triple-positive gliomas?

    (a) *TERT* promoter mutations
    (b) *IDH* mutations

(c) 1p/19q codeletion

(d) *ATRX* mutation

Answer: d

Based on the presence or absence of TERT promoter mutations, IDH mutations, and 1p/19q codeletion, diffuse gliomas are classified into **five molecular groups:**

- Triple-positive
- TERT- and IDH-mutated
- IDH-mutated only
- TERT-mutated only
- Triple-negative

10. The MGMT gene is located in which of the following chromosomes?

    (a) 1
    (b) 3
    (c) 10
    (d) 19

    Answer: c

    - The MGMT gene (chromosome 10) encodes the MGMT protein, which plays a role in repairing the DNA damage from alkylating agents (including temozolomide).
    - Methylation of the MGMT promoter region → silencing of gene expression (40–50% of glioblastomas).
    - The tumors with low MGMT are deficient in repairing the DNA damage induced by TMZ → Higher chemosensitivity.

11. What are the possible grades for an oligodendroglioma that is IDH-mutant, and 1p/19q-codeleted?

    (a) 1, 2
    (b) 2, 3
    (c) 3,4
    (d) 1, 2, 3

    Answer: b

    - Oligodendroglioma, IDH-mutant, and 1p/19q-codeleted can be of grades 2 or 3.

12. What is the grade of diffuse hemispheric glioma?

    (a) 1
    (b) 2
    (c) 3
    (d) 4

    Answer: d

    Diffuse hemispheric glioma, H3 G34-mutant

    - Malignant and infiltrative glioma added to the 2021 WHO classification
    - Typically involves the cerebral hemispheres
    - Caused by a missense mutation in the H3F3A gene → G34R/V substitution of histone H3.

13. Which of the following is false about the polymorphous low-grade neuroepithelial tumor of the young (PLNTY)?

    (a) It is associated with a history of epilepsy in young people
    (b) Shows a diffuse growth pattern
    (c) CD34 immunoreactivity is typically absent
    (d) Shows MAPK pathway-activating genetic abnormalities

    Answer: c

    Polymorphous Low-grade Neuroepithelial Tumor of the Young (PLNTY)

    - Glial neoplasm
    - Associated with a history of epilepsy in young people
    - Shows diffuse growth patterns
    - Presence of oligodendroglioma-like components
    - Calcification present
    - CD34 immunoreactivity strongly present
    - MAPK pathway-activating genetic abnormalities

14. What is the typical location of a myxoid glioneuronal tumor?

    (a) Lateral ventricle
    (b) Third ventricle
    (c) Fourth ventricle
    (d) Thalamus

    Answer: a

    Myxoid glioneuronal tumor

    - Typically arises in the septal region and involves the lateral ventricle
    - Characterized by a proliferation of oligodendrocyte-like tumor cells embedded in a prominent myxoid stroma

- Often includes a mixture of floating neurons, neurocytic rosettes, and/or perivascular neuropil
- Dinucleotide mutation in the PDGFRA gene.

15. Which of the following is false regarding medulloblastomas in the latest WHO classification?

(a) All true desmoplastic/nodular medulloblastomas and MBENs belong to the SHH-1 and SHH-2 subgroups
(b) Nearly all WNT tumors have a classic morphology
(c) Most large cell/anaplastic tumors belong either to the SHH-3 subgroup or to the Group 3/4 subgroup
(d) Nearly all WNT tumors have a large cell/anaplastic morphology

Answer: d

16. Which of the following molecular subtypes of pineoblastoma is associated with a good prognosis?

(a) Pineoblastoma, miRNA processing-altered 1
(b) Pineoblastoma, miRNA processing-altered 2
(c) Pineoblastoma, MYC/FOXR2-activated
(d) Pineoblastoma, RB1-altered

Answer: b

Pineoblastomas—4 molecular subtypes:

- Pineoblastoma, miRNA processing-altered 1

  – Children
  – DICER1, DROSHA, or DGCR8 mutations

- Pineoblastoma, miRNA processing-altered 2

  – Mostly older children
  – Least chance of metastasis
  – Relatively good prognosis
  – DICER1, DROSHA, or DGCR8 mutations

- Pineoblastoma, MYC/FOXR2-activated

  – Infants—males are more prone
  – MYC activation and FOXR2 overexpression

- Pineoblastoma, RB1-altered

  – Infants—females are more prone
  – Similarities to retinoblastoma
  – 100% chance of metastasis

17. Match the following types of meningiomas with their characteristic molecular features/mutations.

(a) SMARCE1	WHO grade 3
(b) BAP1	Secretory subtype
(c) KLF4/TRAF7	Clear cell subtype
(d) TERT promoter	Rhabdoid and papillary subtypes

Answer:

1. SMARCE1	Clear cell subtype
2. BAP1	Rhabdoid and papillary subtypes
3. KLF4/TRAF7	Secretory subtype
4. TERT promoter mutation	WHO grade 3

- H3K27me3 loss of nuclear expression is associated with a worse prognosis in meningiomas

18. Which of the following is false regarding pediatric-type diffuse glioma?

    (a) Shares overlying histology with their adult counterpart
    (b) Generally indolent despite anaplastic histological features
    (c) Characterized by IDH mutation and 1p/19q codeletion
    (d) Usually harbors MAPK-pathway alteration

    Answer: c

    - The genetic hallmark of adult-type gliomas is IDH mutation and 1p/19q codeletion. But pediatric-type diffuse gliomas lack this mutation.

19. Which of the following is not a central nervous system soft tissue tumor of uncertain differentiation?

    (a) Intracranial mesenchymal tumor, FET-CREB fusion-positive
    (b) Rhabdomyosarcoma
    (c) Primary intracranial sarcoma, DICER1-mutant
    (d) Ewing sarcoma

    Answer: b

- **Soft tissue tumors of uncertain differentiation:**
    - Intracranial mesenchymal tumor, FET-CREB fusion-positive
    - CIC-rearranged sarcoma
    - Primary intracranial sarcoma, DICER1-mutant
    - Ewing sarcoma

20. CNS tumor with BCOR internal tandem duplication is included provisionally under which group in the WHO 2021 classification?

    (a) Mesenchymal, non-meningothelial tumors
    (b) Hematolymphoid tumors
    (c) Embryonal tumors
    (d) Glioneuronal and neuronal tumors

    Answer: c

    CNS tumor with BCOR internal tandem duplication

- Mostly solid growth pattern
- Uniform oval or spindle-shaped cells
- Dense capillary network
- Focal pseudorosette formation
- Internal tandem duplication (ITD) in exon 15 of the BCOR gene.

Test your learning and check your understanding of this book's contents: use the "Springer Nature Flashcards" app to access questions. To use the app, please follow the instructions below: 1. Go to https://flashcards.springernature.com/login 2. Create a user account by entering your e-mail address and assigning a password. 3. Use the following link to access your SN Flashcards set: https://sn.pub/3HwHCw If the link is missing or does not work, please send an e-mail with the subject "SN Flashcards".

Bibliography

1. Louis DN, Perry A, Wesseling P, Brat DJ, Cree IA, Figarella-Branger D, Hawkins C, Ng HK, Pfister SM, Reifenberger G, Soffietti R, von Deimling A, Ellison DW. The 2021 WHO classification of tumors of the central nervous system: a summary. Neuro-Oncology. 2021;23(8):1231–51. https://doi.org/10.1093/neuonc/noab106.

Chapter 2
Molecular Genetics and Syndromes

Joe M Das

1. Which of the following is the most common neoplasm of the central nervous system associated with neurofibromatosis type 1?

   (a) Neurofibroma
   (b) Optic pathway glioma
   (c) Optic nerve sheath meningioma
   (d) Sphenoid wing meningioma

   Answer: b

   Optic Pathway Glioma

   - The most common central nervous system tumor seen in patients with NF1.
   - WHO grade 1 pilocytic astrocytoma, histologically.
   - The second most common tumor in the CNS in such patients is a brain stem glioma.

   NF1

   - The most common genetically inherited neurological disorder
   - 1 in 3000 to 4000 live births
   - NF1 tumor suppressor gene (chromosome 17q11.2)
   - Encodes neurofibromin (a cytoplasmic protein) which is a negative regulator of the RAS-MAP kinase pathway involved in cell proliferation.
   - Autosomal dominant
   - 50% of patients may present with de novo mutations
   - Lifetime cancer risk—59.6%

J. M. Das (✉)
Consultant Neurosurgeon, Bahrain Specialist Hospital, Juffair, Bahrain
e-mail: neurosurgeon@doctors.org.uk

- Penetrance is complete, but tumor development cannot be predicted in any one patient.
- Pilocytic astrocytomas are the most common CNS neoplasm associated with NF1.
- In the form of optic pathway glioma (two-thirds of CNS tumors in patients with NF1)
- Leading cause of death—Malignant Peripheral Nerve Sheath Tumors
- Five-fold increased chance for developing glioblastoma
- Intramedullary lesions are more frequently low-grade astrocytomas
- Diagnostic criteria include at least two of the following (NIH):

    (a) Six or more café-au-lait macules with the greatest diameter—>5 mm (pre-pubertal) and >15 mm longest diameter (post-pubertal)
    (b) Two or more neurofibromas or one plexiform neurofibroma
    (c) Intertriginous freckling—axillary or inguinal
    (d) Optic pathway glioma (OPG)
    (e) Two or more iris hamartomas (or Lisch nodules)
    (f) Distinctive osseous lesions (e.g., sphenoid wing dysplasia, thinning of long bones with or without pseudoarthrosis)
    (g) First-degree relative with NF1.

- Screening children with NF1:

    (a) Screening for OPG with yearly comprehensive ophthalmologic evaluation until puberty → Screening every 2 years
    (b) In patients with known lesions, an MRI of the brain (with orbits) with Gd + ophthalmologic evaluation

- Clinical indications for treatment in OPG:

    (a) Progressive visual decline
    (b) Severe exophthalmos
    (c) Precocious puberty
    (d) Radiographic progression

- **Clinical indications for surgery in OPG:** Visual loss, hydrocephalus
- **Treatment of OPG:** Chemotherapy (regimen including carboplatin with vincristine), everolimus
- Five-year survival—90% following chemotherapy
- Extraoptic gliomas (brainstem, diencephalon, cerebellum, or rarely cerebrum):

    (a) Surveillance imaging
    (b) Surgical biopsy if rapid growth
    (c) High grade → Maximal safe resection, radiation, and chemotherapy

- **UBOs:**

    (a) Explanations: hamartomas, altered myelination, or heterotopias
    (b) Vacuoles (5–100 μm) in the myelin sheath and increase of extracellular-like intracellular water correlating to intramyelinic edema.

2. The initial treatment of optic pathway glioma presenting with precocious puberty in a patient with neurofibromatosis type 1 is

   (a) Surgical decompression
   (b) Radiotherapy
   (c) Chemotherapy
   (d) Hormone therapy

   Answer: d

- Clinical indications for treatment in OPG:
    - (a) Progressive visual decline
    - (b) Severe exophthalmos
    - (c) Precocious puberty not responding to hormonal therapy
    - (d) Radiographic progression

- Clinical indication for surgery in OPG: Visual loss, hydrocephalus
- Treatment of OPG: Chemotherapy (regimen including carboplatin with vincristine), everolimus
- Five-year survival—90% following chemotherapy

3. The unidentified bright objects seen in the MRI scan of the craniospinal neuraxis of occasional patients with neurofibromatosis are structurally

   (a) Neurofibromas
   (b) Schwannomas
   (c) Hamartomas
   (d) Intramyelin edema

   Answer: d

   UBOs are derived from

- altered microstructural compartmentalization
- increase in intracellular water
- intramyelinic edema

4. Which of the following is not a major criterion for the diagnosis of tuberous sclerosis?

   (a) Shagreen patch
   (b) Fibrous cephalic plaque
   (c) Retinal hamartoma
   (d) "Confetti" skin lesions

   Answer: d

   Diagnostic Criteria for TSC:

   Dermatologic and dentistry
   Major criteria:

      Hypomelanotic macules (≥3, at least 5 mm diameter)
      Angiofibromas (≥3) or fibrous cephalic plaque

Ungual fibromas (≥2)
Shagreen patch

Minor criteria:

"Confetti" skin lesions
Dental enamel pits (≥3)
Intraoral fibromas (≥2)

Ophthalmologic
Major criterion:

Retinal hamartoma
Minor criterion:

Retinal achromic patch

Brain structure, tubers, and tumors
Major criteria:

Cortical dysplasia
Subependymal nodules
SEGA

Cardiology and pulmonary
Major criteria:

Cardiac rhabdomyoma
LAM

Nephrology
Major criterion:

Angiomyolipomas (≥2)

Minor criterion:

Multiple renal cysts

Other (endocrine, GI)
Minor criterion:

Nonrenal hamartomas

Extra-nervous System Manifestations
Cutaneous angiofibromas, subungual fibromas, cardiac rhabdomyomas, intestinal polyps, visceral cysts, pulmonary lymphangioleiomyomatosis, and renal angiomyolipomas.

Central Nervous System Manifestations

Cortical hamartomas called tubers, subcortical glioneuronal hamartomas, subependymal nodules, and retinal and subependymal giant cell astrocytomas (SEGAs).

5. Which of the following drugs has been approved by the US FDA for the treatment of progressive and inoperable plexiform neurofibromas in symptomatic children?

(a) Trametinib
(b) Cabozantinib
(c) Nilotinib
(d) Selumetinib

Answer: d

- Selumetinib—oral selective inhibitor of mitogen-activated protein kinase (MEK or MAPK/ERK kinase) 1 and 2.
- Indications: Symptomatic children ≥2 years with inoperable and progressive plexiform neurofibromas.

6. Which of the following genetic mutations have been identified as a major determining pathomechanism in Sturge Weber syndrome?

(a) GNAQ
(b) GNAT-1
(c) PIK3CA
(d) ERCC2

Answer: a

Genes Associated with Neurogenetic Syndromes

• Ataxia telangiectasia	ATM (11q22)
• Cowden	PTEN (10q23)
• Gorlin	PTCH1 (9q22), SUFU (10q24)
• Li-Fraumeni	TP53 (17p13)
• Multiple endocrine neoplasia type I	MEN1 (11q13)
• NF-1	Neurofibromin (17q11)
• NF-2	Merlin (22q12)
• Tuberous sclerosis complex	TSC1 (9q34), TSC2 (16q13)
• Turcot	MLH1 (3p22), MSH2 (2p21), PMS2 (7p22), APC (5q21)
• Von Hippel-Lindau syndrome	VHL (3p25)
• Sturge Weber syndrome	GNAQ (9q21)
• Hereditary hemorrhagic telangiectasia	HHT1 (ENG-9q34) and HHT2 (ACVRL1-12q13)
• Rubinstein Taybi syndrome	CREBBP (16p13)
• Melanoma astrocytoma syndrome	CDKN2A (9p21)
• Carney complex	PRKAR1A (17q22–24)
• Rhabdoid tumor predisposition syndrome	SMARCB1 (22q11)
• Melanoma-astrocytoma syndrome	CDKN2A (9p21)
• Retinoblastoma	RB1 (13q14.2)
• Nijmegen breakage syndrome	NBS1 (8q21)

7. Which of the following modalities has shown promise in the treatment of pres-ymptomatic patients with Sturge-Weber syndrome?

    (a) Antiplatelet medications
    (b) Anticonvulsants
    (c) Antiplatelet medications and anticonvulsants
    (d) Observation alone

    Answer: c

    75% of children with brain involvement due to SWS develop seizures in the first year of life.
    Early onset of seizures → poor neurological outcome.
    Treatment to be started at an early age

8. Which of the following is not a major criterion in the diagnosis of Gorlin syndrome?

    (a) Odontogenic keratocysts of the jaw
    (b) Palmar/plantar hyperkeratosis
    (c) Bilamellar calcification of the falx cerebri
    (d) Ovarian or cardiac fibroma

    Answer: d

    Gorlin-Glotz Syndrome

    Major criteria:

    • Basal cell carcinoma <20 years of age
    • Odontogenic keratocysts of the jaws—histologically proven
    • ≥3 Palmar or plantar pits
    • Bilamellar calcification of the falx cerebri
    • First-degree relative with the same syndrome

    Minor criteria:

    • Macrocephaly
    • Cleft lip or palate
    • Hand/feet/rib/vertebral anomalies
    • Ovarian fibroma
    • Medulloblastoma

    2 major +1 minor OR 1 major +3 minor criteria are necessary to establish a diagnosis.

9. Curaçao clinical criteria are used in the diagnosis of which neurocutaneous syndrome?

    (a) Hereditary hemorrhagic telangiectasia
    (b) Gorlin syndrome

(c) Tuberous sclerosis
(d) Sturge Weber syndrome

Answer: a

Curaçao Diagnostic Criteria for HHT (Osler-Weber-Rendu Syndrome)

- Spontaneous and recurrent epistaxis
- Multiple telangiectases— lips, oral cavity, fingers, nose
- Visceral vascular lesions—gastrointestinal telangiectasia; pulmonary, cerebral, hepatic, spinal AVMs
- Family history—first-degree relative with HHT

Three or more criteria to be present for the diagnosis.

10. What is the most common presenting symptom in HHT?

    (a) Bleeding port-wine stain
    (b) Epistaxis
    (c) Hemoptysis
    (d) Melena

    Answer: b

    Epistaxis is the most common symptom that brings a patient with HHT to medical attention.

11. Infantile spasms in tuberous sclerosis can be effectively treated with which of the following medicines?

    (a) Lamotrigine
    (b) Levetiracetam
    (c) Vigabatrin
    (d) Topiramate

    Answer: c

    Oral ganaxolone—phase III evaluation in the treatment of tuberous sclerosis complex-related epilepsy.

12. The genetic cause of Gorlin syndrome is a mutation in the gene located in which of the following chromosomes?

    (a) 9p
    (b) 9q
    (c) 14p
    (d) 14q

    Answer: b

13. Which of the following tumor syndromes is less likely to have an association with medulloblastoma formation?

    (a) Gorlin syndrome
    (b) Ataxia-telangiectasia
    (c) Li-Fraumeni syndrome
    (d) Cowden syndrome

    Answer: d

    The syndromes usually associated with medulloblastoma are

- Gorlin syndrome (nevoid basal cell carcinoma)
- Li Fraumeni syndrome
- Turcot syndrome
- Rubinsten-Taybi syndrome
- Nijmegen breakage syndrome (NBS1 gene—chromosome 8q21)
- Neurofibromatosis
- Ataxia-telangiectasia

14. The NF-1 mutation is located on locus 17q.11.2 which encodes neurofibromin. What is the normal function of this protein?

    (a) Inhibition of the mTOR pathway
    (b) Activation of the mTOR pathway
    (c) Accelerates the inactivation of Ras
    (d) Accelerates the activation of Ras

    Answer: c

- The most common tumor-predisposing disease in humans—NF1
- *NF1* gene—17q11.2 locus
- Neurofibromin—Tumor suppressor protein
- Neurofibromin = GTPase-activating protein of Ras (Ras-GAP) → increases the intrinsic GTPase activity of Ras → promotes the hydrolysis of the active form of Ras (GTP-bound Ras) to an inactive form of Ras (GDP-bound Ras) → downregulates the Ras signaling pathway

15. Which is the most common intramedullary spinal cord tumor associated with NF-2?

    (a) Astrocytoma
    (b) Schwannoma
    (c) Ependymoma
    (d) Ganglioglioma

    Answer: c

    NF2:

- Autosomal dominant
- 1 in 33,000 to 40,000 live births

- NF2 tumor suppressor gene (chromosome 22q12)
- Encodes merlin (Moesin-ezrin-radixin-like protein) or schwannomin (a cytoplasmic protein) which is an enzyme involved in linking membrane-associated proteins to the actin cytoskeleton
- Acts through Ras/Rac/PAK cell proliferation pathway
- Complete penetrance—50% of patients will harbor de novo mutations
- **Clinical Criteria:**

1. Bilateral VIII nerve masses seen with appropriate imaging (CT or MRI) OR First-degree relative with NF-2
   AND
2. Either: Unilateral VIII nerve mass, OR

Two of the following:

(i) Neurofibroma
(ii) Meningioma
(iii) Glioma
(iv) Schwannoma
(v) Juvenile posterior subcapsular lenticular opacity

- Dermal tumors are typically schwannomas.
- Bilateral VS (WHO grade I) are pathognomonic for NF2.
- Collision tumors are composed of both meningioma and schwannoma.
- Initial evaluation of a patient with confirmed or suspected NF2:

  - Comprehensive history and physical examination
  - Audiometry including pure tone threshold and word recognition
  - MRI of the brain with axial and coronal fine cuts through the auditory canal (3-mm slice thickness)
  - MRI of the cervical spine to evaluate for spinal ependymoma.
  - A baseline ophthalmologic examination to assess for posterior subcapsular cataracts (the juvenile form being pathognomonic for NF2)

Surveillance:

- Neuroimaging of suspicious lesions and audiometry every 6 months
- Patients with VS—annual neuroimaging with fine cuts through the internal auditory canal and audiometry.

Goals of treatment:

- Preservation of function—hearing
- Maximizing quality of life.

Causes of hearing loss:

- Vestibular nerve compression
- Cochlear aperture obstruction
- Intralabyrinthine protein accumulation
- Primary hair cell dysfunction

Bilateral VS arise from the superior and inferior vestibular branches of the eighth cranial nerve.

There is no consensus on the management of VS Less than 3 cm—Surgery vs SRS.

Indications for Surgery:

1. Tumor >3 cm
2. Brainstem compression or hydrocephalus
3. Patients not interested in SRS

Drug shown to be effective in the management of NF2-associated VS—Bevacizumab.

Surgery for NF2 meningiomas—Rapid tumor growth or symptomatic neurological decline.

Spinal ependymomas have an indolent course and are typically observed.

16. Which of the following genetic syndromes is associated with Lhermitte- Duclos disease?

    (a) Gorlin syndrome
    (b) Ataxia-telangiectasia
    (c) Li-Fraumeni syndrome
    (d) Cowden syndrome

    Answer: d

17. Which of the following is the least common central nervous system tumor associated with Li-Fraumeni syndrome?

    (a) Choroid plexus carcinoma
    (b) Medulloblastoma
    (c) Astrocytoma
    (d) Ependymoma

    Answer: d

18. Which of the following are the most common brain tumors associated with Li-Fraumeni syndrome?

    (a) Choroid plexus carcinoma
    (b) Medulloblastoma
    (c) Astrocytoma
    (d) Ependymoma

    Answer: c

19. What is the first-line treatment for subependymal giant cell astrocytoma associated with tuberous sclerosis?

    (a) Mammalian target of rapamycin inhibitor
    (b) Surgical excision

(c) Radiotherapy

(d) Laser therapy

Answer: a

20. The most common genetic mutation in Rubinstein-Taybi syndrome is in which of the following genes?

(a) CREBBP

(b) C-MYB

(c) C-FOS

(d) CITED2

Answer: a

21. Which is the most common type of pituitary adenoma associated with Multiple Endocrine Neoplasia type 1?

(a) Growth Hormone adenoma

(b) Non-functioning adenoma

(c) Corticotroph adenoma

(d) Prolactinoma

Answer: d

22. Which CNS tumor is most commonly associated with Turcot syndrome 1?

(a) Meningioma

(b) Hemangioblastoma

(c) Medulloblastoma

(d) Glioma

Answer: d

Test your learning and check your understanding of this book's contents: use the "Springer Nature Flashcards" app to access questions using https://sn.pub/3HwHCw To use the app, please follow the instructions in Chap. 1.

Bibliography

1. Billiet T, Mädler B, D'Arco F, Peeters R, Deprez S, Plasschaert E, Leemans A, Zhang H, den Bergh BV, Vandenbulcke M, Legius E, Sunaert S, Emsell L. Characterizing the microstructural basis of "unidentified bright objects" in neurofibromatosis type 1: a combined in vivo multicomponent T2 relaxation and multi-shell diffusion MRI analysis. Neuroimage Clin. 2014;13(4):649–58. https://doi.org/10.1016/j.nicl.2014.04.005.
2. Amaravathi A, Oblinger JL, Welling DB, Kinghorn AD, Chang LS. Neurofibromatosis: molecular pathogenesis and natural compounds as potential treatments. Front Oncol. 2021;17(11):698192. https://doi.org/10.3389/fonc.2021.698192.

3. Day AM, Hammill AM, Juhász C, Pinto AL, Roach ES, CE MC, Comi AM, National Institutes of Health Sponsor: Rare Diseases Clinical Research Network (RDCRN) Brain and Vascular Malformation Consortium (BVMC) SWS Investigator Group. Hypothesis: Presymptomatic treatment of Sturge-weber syndrome with aspirin and antiepileptic drugs may delay seizure onset. Pediatr Neurol. 2019;90:8–12. https://doi.org/10.1016/j.pediatrneurol.2018.04.009. Epub 2018 Nov 24

4. Yum MS, Lee EH, Ko TS. Vigabatrin and mental retardation in tuberous sclerosis: infantile spasms versus focal seizures. J Child Neurol. 2013;28(3):308–13. https://doi.org/10.1177/0883073812446485. Epub 2012 Jun 29

5. Jawa DS, Sircar K, Somani R, Grover N, Jaidka S, Singh S. Gorlin-Goltz syndrome. J Oral Maxillofac Pathol. 2009;13(2):89–92. https://doi.org/10.4103/0973-029X.57677.

6. McDonald J, Bayrak-Toydemir P, DeMille D, Wooderchak-Donahue W, Whitehead K. Curaçao diagnostic criteria for hereditary hemorrhagic telangiectasia is highly predictive of a pathogenic variant in ENG or ACVRL1 (HHT1 and HHT2). Genet Med. 2020;22(7):1201–5. https://doi.org/10.1038/s41436-020-0775-8. Epub 2020 Apr 17

7. Garg N, Khunger M, Gupta A, Kumar N. Optimal management of hereditary hemorrhagic telangiectasia. J Blood Med. 2014;15(5):191–206. https://doi.org/10.2147/JBM.S45295.

8. Carta R, Del Baldo G, Miele E, Po A, Besharat ZM, Nazio F, Colafati GS, Piccirilli E, Agolini E, Rinelli M, Lodi M, Cacchione A, Carai A, Boccuto L, Ferretti E, Locatelli F, Mastronuzzi A. Cancer predisposition syndromes and Medulloblastoma in the molecular era. Front Oncol. 2020;29(10):566822. https://doi.org/10.3389/fonc.2020.566822.

9. Bergoug M, Doudeau M, Godin F, Mosrin C, Vallée B, Bénédetti H. Neurofibromin structure, functions and regulation. Cell. 2020;9(11):2365. https://doi.org/10.3390/cells9112365.

Chapter 3
Angiogenesis

Joe M Das

1. Match the following genes with the corresponding property related to angiogenesis

   (a) Angiogenesis promoter
   (b) Angiogenesis inhibitor

      i. VEGF
      ii. HGF-SF
      iii. bFGF
      iv. Angiopoietin 2
      v. Interferon-α
      vi. IL-6
      vii. TIMP 1

   Answer:

• Angiogenesis promoters	VEGF, HGF-SF, bFGF, IL-6
• Angiogenesis inhibitors	Angiopoietin 2, interferon-α, TIMP 1

   • Other important proangiogenic factors include CXCL12 (SDF1α), HIF1α, angiopoietin 1, TGF-β1, IL-1a, IL-6, and IL-8.
   • Other important proangiogenic factors include CXCL12 (SDF1α), HIF1α, angiopoietin 1, TGF-β1, IL-1a, IL-6, and IL-8.
      ? Cause → Hypoxia → Release of proangiogenic factors (PAF) → Binding of PAF with receptors on the endothelial cell membrane → Dissolution of the blood vessel wall → Degradation of the endothelial cell basement membrane and ECM → Remodeling the ECM components by MMP → Stromal

J. M. Das (✉)
Consultant Neurosurgeon, Bahrain Specialist Hospital, Juffair, Bahrain
e-mail: neurosurgeon@doctors.org.uk

J. M. Das, *Neuro-Oncology Explained Through Multiple Choice Questions*, https://doi.org/10.1007/978-3-031-13253-7_3

cells create new matrix → migration and proliferation of endothelial cells → endothelial tube-like structure → a mature vascular basement membrane is formed around this → Mural cells (pericytes and smooth muscle cells) surrounding it resulting in a stable new vessel.

2. Which of the following is the main mediator in hypoxia-induced tumor growth?

(a) VEGF A
(b) VEGF B
(c) VEGF C
(d) VEGF D

Answer: a

- Overexpression of VEGF and VEGF-R1 in the low-grade astrocytomas → dismal prognosis like high-grade lesions.
- VEGF-A is the most potent angiogenic factor (gene located on the short arm of chromosome six)

3. Which of the following MMPs are highly expressed in patients with WHO grade 3 brain tumors?

(a) MMP 1 and 2
(b) MMP 2 and 9
(c) MMP 4 and 9
(d) MMP 1 and 4

Answer: b

- Gelatinase-A (MMP-2) and gelatinase-B (MMP-9) are highly expressed in patients with WHO grade 3 brain tumors

4. Match the following therapeutic agents with their molecular targets:

(a) Cilengitide	HIF 1A
(b) Bevacizumab	VEGFR2, EGFR
(c) Panzem®	Integrins $\alpha\nu\beta3$ and $\alpha\nu\beta5$
(d) Vandetanib	VEGF A

Answer:

1. Cilengitide	Integrins $\alpha\nu\beta3$ and $\alpha\nu\beta5$
2. Bevacizumab	VEGF A
3. Panzem®	HIF 1A
4. Vandetanib	VEGFR2, EGFR

5. Which of the following is false regarding Bevacizumab?

(a) It is approved for use in recurrent glioblastoma in the US
(b) The usual dose is 15–20 mg/kg
(c) Mild epistaxis is the most common form of bleeding seen as a side effect
(d) Hypertension is one of the most commonly seen side effects

Answer: b

6. Which of the following molecules is being tried to overcome resistance to bevacizumab by cancer cells?

   (a) Nintedanib
   (b) Sunitinib
   (c) Sorafenib
   (d) Pazopanib

   Answer: a

   Nintedanib (BIBF 1120): triple angiokinase (tyrosine kinase) inhibitor
   (inhibitor of VEGFR, PDGFR, and FGFR)

7. Which of the following anti-parasitic agent has been used as a low-toxicity
   treatment against angiogenesis in medulloblastoma?

   (a) Hydroxychloroquine
   (b) Albendazole
   (c) Mebendazole
   (d) Ivermectin

   Answer: c

8. Which of the following viruses can promote all the stages of angiogenesis and
   is considered a target for the treatment of glioblastoma?

   (a) Human immunodeficiency virus
   (b) Cytomegalovirus
   (c) Herpes simplex virus
   (d) JC virus

   Answer: b

9. Which type of glioblastoma has shown the maximum response to anti-
   angiogenic treatment?

   (a) IDH1 wild-type, proneural glioblastoma
   (b) IDH1 mutant, proneural glioblastoma
   (c) IDH1 wild-type, proliferative glioblastoma
   (d) IDH1 mutant, proliferative glioblatoma

   Answer: a

10. Match the following therapeutic agents with their mechanism of action:

(a) Bevacizumab: Inhibitor of mTOR.
(b) Aflibercept: Inhibitor of PI3K pathway
(c) Sunitinib: Binds to VEGF A and renders it unavailable to bind to receptors
(d) Sorafenib: Prevents binding of VEGF-A to receptors
(e) Wortmannin: Tyrosine kinase inhibitor
(f) Everolimus: Inhibits MAPK signaling
(g) Lonafarnib: Inhibitor of intracellular Raf kinase and targets MAPK, Raf/MEK/ERK signaling pathways

Answer:

(a) Bevacizumab: Prevents binding of VEGF-A to receptors.
(b) Aflibercept: Binds to VEGF A and renders it unavailable to bind to receptors
(c) Sunitinib: Tyrosine kinase inhibitor
(d) Sorafenib: Inhibitor of intracellular Raf kinase and targets MAPK, Raf/MEK/ERK signaling pathways
(e) Wortmannin: Inhibitor of PI3K pathway
(f) Everolimus: Inhibitor of mTOR.
(g) Lonafarnib: Inhibits MAPK signaling

11. Which of the following microRNAs is most important in the intercellular communication from glioblastoma to endothelial cells and astrocytes?

    (a) miR-21
    (b) miR-301a
    (c) miR-124-3p
    (d) miR-5096

    Answer: d

12. Glioma cells move towards and along the pre-existing tissue blood vessels and utilize them to support tumor growth, survival, and metastasis. What is this process known as?

    (a) Angiogenic switch
    (b) Vessel co-option
    (c) Vasculogenic mimicry
    (d) Intussusception

    Answer: b

    Angiogenic switch:

    - It is a time-restricted event during tumor progression.
    - The balance between pro- and anti-angiogenic factors favors a pro-angiogenic outcome during this event.
    - This results in the transition: Dormant avascularized hyperplasia → Vascularized tumor → Malignant tumor progression.

    Key steps:

    - Gene mutation / Hypoxia → Glioma cells release VEGF / bFGF → Activate brain endothelial cells (Switch event) → Angiogenic phenotype.
    - VEGF binds to endothelial cell receptors → Activate signal transduction pathways → Endothelial cell proliferation
    - Sprouting vessels → Urokinase and MMPs → Vessels migrate toward the tumor using $\alpha\beta$ integrins.

    Vessel Co-option

    - Glioma cells surround the host vessels → Migration along these vessels away from the main tumor mass → Protected environment (vascular niche)

- The critical size of the glioma cluster 5×10^5 cells $\rightarrow$ Recruitment of its own additional vessels $\rightarrow$ The process is repeated

Vasculogenic mimicry

- Tumor cells $\rightarrow$ trans-differentiation $\rightarrow$ Obtain features of endothelial cells $\rightarrow$ Form vessel-like structures lacking endothelium $\rightarrow$ Connect with blood vessels to supply blood to the tumor.

Intussusception (Intussusceptive or Splitting Angiogenesis)

- Formation of new blood vessels by splitting off existing vessels. The capillary wall extends into the single blood vessel lumen in two.

Angiotherapy

- Decreasing the tumor volume by inhibiting angiogenesis

Vasculogenesis

- Differentiation of precursor cells (angioblasts) or bone marrow−derived cells $\rightarrow$ Endothelial cells $\rightarrow$ Formation of a primitive vascular network

Angiogenesis

- The proliferation of endothelial cells from local preexisting vessels.

13. Bevacizumab is not approved by FDA in the treatment of

   (a) Metastatic colorectal cancer
   (b) Metastatic renal cell cancer
   (c) Newly diagnosed glioblastoma
   (d) Recurrent glioblastoma

   Answer: c

14. Which is not a histological pattern of secondary structures of Scherer?

   (a) Subpial spread
   (b) Perineuronal satellitosis
   (c) Perivascular satellitosis
   (d) Subarachnoid spread

   Answer: d

   Secondary Structures of Scherer

   The glioma cells migrate away from the main tumor mass through the brain parenchyma. These are called secondary structures of Scherer.
   Four types of spread:

- Subpial spread
- Perineuronal satellitosis
- Perivascular satellitosis
- Invasion along white matter tracts

15. Which of the following markers and their receptors are expressed by most of the different cell types of the glioblastoma microenvironment?

   (a) DCC
   (b) NEO1
   (c) Netrin-1
   (d) UNC5

   Answer: c

Test your learning and check your understanding of this book's contents: use the "Springer Nature Flashcards" app to access questions using https://sn.pub/3HwHCw To use the app, please follow the instructions in Chap. 1.

Bibliography

1. Buruiană A, Florian ŞI, Florian AI, Timiş TL, Mihu CM, Miclăuş M, Oşan S, Hrapşa I, Cataniciu RC, Farcaş M, Şuşman S. The roles of miRNA in Glioblastoma tumor cell communication: diplomatic and aggressive negotiations. Int J Mol Sci. 2020;21(6):1950. https://doi.org/10.3390/ijms21061950.
2. Hara A, Kanayama T, Noguchi K, Niwa A, Miyai M, Kawaguchi M, Ishida K, Hatano Y, Niwa M, Tomita H. Treatment strategies based on histological targets against invasive and resistant Glioblastoma. J Oncol. 2019;2019:2964783. https://doi.org/10.1155/2019/2964783.
3. Vásquez X, Sánchez-Gómez P, Palma V. Netrin-1 in Glioblastoma neovascularization: the new partner in crime? Int J Mol Sci. 2021;22(15):8248. https://doi.org/10.3390/ijms22158248.

Chapter 4
Epidemiology

Joe M Das

1. Which of the following factors is not associated with better survival in patients with glioblastoma?

   (a) IDH mutation
   (b) Less contrast enhancement on MRI scan
   (c) Young age
   (d) Involvement of splenium

   Answer: d

   The variables associated with better prognosis of glioblastoma:

   - Younger age
   - *IDH* mutation in the tumor
   - Higher Karnofsky Performance Scale score
   - Greater extent of resection and capacity for complete resection
   - Lower degree of tumor necrosis
   - Less contrast enhancement in the tumor on preoperative magnetic resonance imaging studies
   - Decreased volume of residual disease
   - Smaller preoperative and postoperative tumor size
   - More favorable tumor location (poorer survival is associated with tumor infiltration of the splenium, basal ganglia, thalamus, or midbrain)

J. M. Das (✉)
Consultant Neurosurgeon, Bahrain Specialist Hospital, Juffair, Bahrain
e-mail: neurosurgeon@doctors.org.uk

© The Author(s), under exclusive license to Springer Nature Switzerland AG 2023
J. M. Das, *Neuro-Oncology Explained Through Multiple Choice Questions*,
https://doi.org/10.1007/978-3-031-13253-7_4

2. Match the following mutations with the glioblastoma subtype in which they are commonly seen.

(a) Classical	SLC12A
(b) Mesenchymal	EGFR amplification
(c) Proneural	Hemizygous deletion of NF1
(d) Proneural	PDGFRA mutation

Answer:

Classical	EGFR amplification
Mesenchymal	Hemizygous deletion of NF1
Proneural	PDGFRA mutation
Neural	SLC12A5

3. Which is the familial tumor syndrome most frequently associated with glioma?

   (a) Li-Fraumeni syndrome
   (b) Multiple endocrine neoplasia—I
   (c) Multiple endocrine neoplasia—II
   (d) Neurofibromatosis—1

   Answer: a

4. Which single nucleotide polymorphism (SNP) is associated with a six-fold increased risk of developing an *IDH*-mutant glioma?

   (a) 8q24.21 SNP
   (b) 8p24.21 SNP
   (c) 10q21.24 SNP
   (d) 10p21.24 SNP

   Answer: a

5. Which of the following interleukins present in allergic conditions reduce the risk of gliomagenesis?

   (a) IL-1 and IL-3
   (b) IL-2 and IL-14
   (c) IL-3 and IL-8
   (d) IL-4 and IL-13

   Answer: d

6. Smoking has been inversely related to the risk of development of which of the following tumors?

   (a) Low-grade glioma
   (b) High-grade glioma
   (c) Meningioma
   (d) Acoustic neuroma

   Answer: d

7. Which of the following is the most common type of secondary brain tumor following cranial radiotherapy?

   (a) Low-grade glioma
   (b) High-grade glioma
   (c) Meningioma
   (d) Acoustic neuroma

   Answer: c

8. Which of the following cancers is the most common primary to be identified in a patient with CNS metastasis?

   (a) Lung and bronchus
   (b) Breast
   (c) Melanoma
   (d) Kidney

   Answer: a

9. Which of the following countries/continents has the lowest mortality due to brain tumors?

   (a) United States of America
   (b) United Kingdom
   (c) Australia
   (d) Japan

   Answer: d

10. What is the position of brain tumors in the hierarchical order of average years of life lost due to the disease?

    (a) First
    (b) Second
    (c) Third
    (d) Fourth

    Answer: d

    Testes, cervix, and Hodgkin Lymphoma occupy the first, second, and third positions respectively.

11. Which of the following tumors has the highest rate of CNS metastasis among all cancer types?

    (a) Lung and bronchus
    (b) Breast
    (c) Melanoma
    (d) Kidney

    Answer: c

12. World Brain Tumor Day is celebrated on

    (a) April 11
    (b) June 8
    (c) October 25
    (d) October 29

    Answer: b

    • April 11—World Parkinson Disease Day
    • October 25—World Spina Bifida and Hydrocephalus Day
    • October 29—World Stroke Day

13. Worldwide age-standardized annual incidence of primary malignant brain tumors is

    (a) 1.3 per 100,000 males
    (b) 2.6 per 100,000 males
    (c) 3.9 per 100,000 males
    (d) 4.8 per 100,000 males

    Answer: c

    • Worldwide age-standardized annual incidence of primary malignant brain tumors is:

        – ~3.9 per 100,000 for males
        – ~3 per 100,000 for females

    • Worldwide age-standardized mortality of primary malignant brain tumors is:

        – ~3.2 per 100,000 for males
        – ~2.4 per 100,000 for females

14. Which of the following statements regarding brain tumors is false?

    (a) Most malignant primary brain tumors occurring in the cerebral cortex develop in the frontal lobe
    (b) Brain malignancy contributes to the fourth highest number of years of life lost due to cancer
    (c) Mortality rates in some Asian countries are lower due to brain cancer when compared to Western countries
    (d) Up to 50% of people with primary cancers in other parts of the body will develop metastases to the brain

    Answer: d

    Up to 30% of people with primary cancers in other parts of the body will develop metastases to the brain.

15. Which of the following is a protective factor against pediatric brain tumors?

    (a) Male sex
    (b) Non-Hispanic/White ethnicity
    (c) Parental age
    (d) Early life exposure to infections

    Answer: d

    Risk Factors:

    • Ionizing radiation
    • Hereditary cancer syndromes
    • Birth defects
    • Male sex
    • Non-Hispanic/White ethnicity
    • Paternal age and high socioeconomic status
    • Dietary N-nitroso compounds
    • High birth weight

    Allergic and atopic conditions are protective factors.

Test your learning and check your understanding of this book's contents: use the "Springer Nature Flashcards" app to access questions using https://sn.pub/3HwHCw To use the app, please follow the instructions in Chap. 1.

Bibliography

1. Oktay Y, Ülgen E, Can Ö, Akyerli CB, Yüksel Ş, Erdemgil Y, Durası IM, Henegariu OI, Nanni EP, Selevsek N, Grossmann J, Erson-Omay EZ, Bai H, Gupta M, Lee W, Turcan Ş, Özpınar A, Huse JT, Sav MA, Flanagan A, Günel M, Sezerman OU, Yakıcıer MC, Pamir MN, Özduman K. IDH-mutant glioma specific association of rs55705857 located at 8q24.21 involves MYC deregulation. Sci Rep. 2016;10(6):27569. https://doi.org/10.1038/srep27569.
2. Gould J. Breaking down the epidemiology of brain cancer. Nature. 2018;561(7724):S40–1. https://doi.org/10.1038/d41586-018-06704-7.
3. Tawbi H, To TM, Bartley K, Sadetsky N, Burton E, Haydu L, McKenna E. Treatment patterns and clinical outcomes for patients with melanoma and central nervous system metastases: a real-world study. Cancer Med. 2022;11(1):139–50. https://doi.org/10.1002/cam4.4438. Epub 2021 Dec 7
4. Sung H, Ferlay J, Siegel RL, Laversanne M, Soerjomataram I, Jemal A, Bray F. Global cancer statistics 2020: GLOBOCAN estimates of incidence and mortality worldwide for 36 cancers in 185 countries. CA Cancer J Clin. 2021;71(3):209–49. https://doi.org/10.3322/caac.21660. Epub 2021 Feb 4
5. Adel Fahmideh M, Scheurer ME. Pediatric brain tumors: descriptive epidemiology, risk factors, and future directions. Cancer Epidemiol Biomark Prev. 2021;30(5):813–21. https://doi.org/10.1158/1055-9965.EPI-20-1443. Epub 2021 Mar 2

Chapter 5
White Matter Fiber Tracts

Dia R. Halalmeh and Marc D. Moisi

1. A 54-year-old man is being evaluated for muscle weakness. The patient drinks alcohol daily and has been binge drinking for the past 2 days. He has had no numbness, vision changes, or dizziness. The patient's only other medical condition is hypertension for which he takes captopril and chlorthalidone. This morning, the patient stumbled and fell several times while trying to get to the bathroom. Physical examination shows right lower extremity weakness but sensation to touch and vibration is normal. MRI was performed and revealed 2 cm × 4 cm irregular lesion in the left hemisphere with mild midline shift. A diagnosis of glioblastoma multiforme was made and surgical resection was recommended. Over the 2 weeks following surgery, the patient gradually developed slurred speech and his wife, who accompanied him, says "he sounds like a robot when he speaks". Diffusion tractography would show disruption to which of the following white matter tracts in this patient?

   (a) Corticospinal tract
   (b) Inferior longitudinal fasciculus
   (c) Superior longitudinal fasciculus (branch III)
   (d) Optic radiation
   (e) Arcuate fasciculus

   Answer: c

   This patient's speech difficulty manifesting as slurred, robot-like speech is consistent with **acquired dysarthria**. In the context of surgical resection of a brain tumor (glioblastoma in this case), his symptoms are most likely due to damage to a key pathway involved in the motor articulatory aspect of speech. Of the given choices, **superior longitudinal fasciculus (branch III)** (SLF) is

D. R. Halalmeh (✉) · M. D. Moisi
Department of Neurosurgery, Hurley Medical Center, Flint, MI, USA
e-mail: dya0120048@med.ju.edu.jo

© The Author(s), under exclusive license to Springer Nature Switzerland AG 2023
J. M. Das, *Neuro-Oncology Explained Through Multiple Choice Questions*,
https://doi.org/10.1007/978-3-031-13253-7_5

the most likely correct answer. SLF is a recently discovered association tract located laterally to the centrum semiovale and typically connects the pars opercularis and inferior portion of premotor cortex to supramarginal gyrus. Damage to any of these components usually results in dysarthric or anarthric speech. Therefore, diffusion tractography (DT) has been investigated in many studies to predict recovery of postoperative language deficits. Preservation of parietotemporal and arcuate fibers (part of the SLF) has been associated with preserved language postoperatively.

Points to remember

The Superior Longitudinal Fasciculus represents a major association tract that links the pars operculum in the frontal lobe to the supramarginal gyrus in the parietal lobe. Damage to this white matter tract can result in dysarthria or anarthria. Early postoperative diffusion tractography facilitates the evaluation of SLF integrity along with its associated fibers, and therefore, the prognosis of language preservation and recovery can be easily predicted.

2. A 62-year-old, right-handed woman is brought to the emergency department by her husband due to confusion. This morning, the husband found her confused and disoriented on the bed. She had also urinated on herself. Temperature is 36.8 °C (98.2 F), blood pressure is 140/84 mm Hg, pulse is 92/min, and respirations are 20/min. Oxygen saturation is 96% on room air. On physical examination, the patient is somnolent but rouses to voice. Pupils are equal and briskly reactive. There is no facial droop, but a small laceration on the lateral border of the tongue is present. MRI imaging demonstrates a large infiltrative tumor involving the corpus callosum and right middle frontal gyrus, and does not enhance with contrast. The patient undergoes frontoparietal craniotomy. Which of the following imaging modalities will be most useful in maximizing tumor resection while minimizing injury to subcortical tracts and structures prior to the surgery?

(a) Computed tomography (CT) with contrast
(b) Computed tomography (CT) without contrast
(c) Fluid-attenuated inversion recovery (FLAIR)
(d) Diffusion tensor (DT) imaging
(e) Functional magnetic resonance imaging (fMRI)
(f) Short Tau Inversion Recovery (STIR) imaging

Answer: d

This patient with an infiltrative brain tumor (as seen in MRI) developed a seizure (evidenced by urinary incontinence and lateral tongue biting in this patient). This is a common initial presentation for most infiltrative cerebral neoplasms. In many patients, surgical resection is typically recommended. However, surgical planning and postoperative potential complications should be discussed with the patient. The risks of adverse outcomes should be weighed against the benefit of adequate surgical resection. This is usually a challenging issue that encounters most neurosurgeons when making the final physician-patient shared decision, particularly in a patient with infiltrative lesions.

Therefore, a variety of imaging modalities have been developed to facilitate the delicate identification of the long white matter tracts within the brain parenchyma. Of these, **diffusion tensor (DT) imaging**, a diffusion-weighted (DW)-based neuroimaging, has been successfully used to map white matter tracts in the brain and to delineate anatomical directions of these tracts that otherwise cannot be identified using the standard functional MRI. Furthermore, the integrity of such tracts can be easily characterized using color-coded DT maps.

Points to remember

Detailed anatomical characterization of white matter tracts as well as evaluating the integrity of these pathways minimize injury associated with surgical resection and help improves postoperative outcomes and recovery. Diffusion Tensor (DT) mapping is a useful tool for surgical planning in patients with infiltrative brain tumors.

3. A 58-year-old Hispanic male presents to the office due to gradually worsening headaches and changes in concentration. The patient developed these headaches a month ago and since then has had continuous throbbing pain over the left side of his head that is associated with nausea. He has had no trauma, neck stiffness, fever, double or blurry vision, or photophobia. The patient appears diaphoretic and uncomfortable on examination. Blood pressure is 130/75 mm Hg and pulse is 110/min. Neurological examination is unremarkable. A non-contrast head CT scan revealed a bihemispheric hypodense lesion crossing the midline to the contralateral parietal lobe with surrounding edema. Direct extension along which of the following white matter tracts most likely explains this patient's radiographic appearance?

(a) Corona radiata
(b) Optic radiation
(c) Fornix
(d) Acoustic radiation
(e) Commissural fibers
(f) Uncinate fascicle

Answer: e

This patient's presenting symptoms and radiographic findings are consistent with an expanding intracranial neoplasm. The presence of an intra-axial heterogenous mass with bilateral cerebral hemisphere involvement is highly suggestive of glioblastoma multiforme, the most common primary brain tumor in adults. This "butterfly" configuration is most commonly due to direct extension along the corpus callosum. The **corpus callosum** (the largest white matter in the brain) is composed of a bundle of **commissural subcortical fibers** connecting the two hemispheres and allowing for rapid communication. It is typically resistant to infiltration except for aggressive tumors such as grade 4 astrocytoma (glioblastoma multiforme). Therefore, any lesion across the midline should raise suspicion for glioblastoma.

Points to remember

Clinicians should have a high index of suspicion with a low threshold for investigation of suspected glioblastoma multiforme. The aggressive tumor is notorious for its involvement of both cerebral hemispheres by direct extension along the corpus callosum; normally an infiltration-resistant subcortical structure.

4. A daughter brings her 69-year-old mother to the office for evaluation of her facial appearance. She reports that she woke up this morning with unusually excessive saliva on her pillow. Her medical history is notable for poorly controlled, long-standing hypertension and diabetes mellitus. Medications include aspirin, metoprolol, valsartan, hydrochlorothiazide, amlodipine, atorvastatin, and metformin. She has a 20-pack-year smoking history but quit 8 years ago. The patient is retired and lives with her only daughter. Blood pressure is 177/100 mm Hg in the left arm and 180/100 mm Hg in the right. A focused neurological examination shows right-sided weakness in the upper extremity that is most noticeable in the hand as well as facial asymmetry. She has no difficulty closing her eyes tight, however, drooping of the right corner of the mouth on the right side is noted. Which of the following fibers subtypes is most likely affected in this patient?

   (a) Commissural fibers
   (b) Projection fibers
   (c) Association fibers
   (d) Cerebellopontine fibers
   (e) Optic pathway

Answer: b

This patient presents with acute, focal neurologic deficits, which should raise concern for stroke. The presence of unilateral facial symptoms along with sparing of the forehead is consistent with an upper motor neuron lesion of the connection from the motor cortex to the facial nucleus in the pons.

Based on their connectivity, white matter tracts are typically classified into projection, association, and commissural fibers. The **projection fibers** connect the cortical grey matter with subcortical structures (eg, basal ganglia, head and face nuclei in the brain stem, cerebellum, and spinal cord). The **corticobulbar tract**, part of the projection white matter fibers, generally provides upper motor control of the contralateral brain stem nuclei, except for the facial and hypoglossal nuclei which receive bilateral input from both hemispheres. In this patient, the anterior limb (ie corticospinal tract, explaining her right-sided weakness) and genu (corticobulbar tract, explaining her facial palsy) of the internal capsule are most likely affected by the stroke.

Points to remember

White matter tracts are classified into three fiber bands based on their connectivity: projection, association, and commissural fibers. Projection fibers represent tracts between the grey matter and subcortical structures.

5. A 51-year-old woman comes to the clinic for recurrent seizures. After evaluation, she is diagnosed with WHO grade 2 "Diffuse" astrocytoma. The neurosurgeon discusses surgical removal with the patient and informed consent was obtained. Due to the infiltrative nature of the tumor, the surgeon bilaterally resects part of the posterior fibers of the inferior longitudinal fasciculus (ILF) tract. Based on the above information, which of the following is most likely to result from this patient's surgical intervention?

   (a) Dysarthria
   (b) Pure alexia
   (c) Hearing loss
   (d) Aphasia
   (e) Paresis
   (f) Hypertonia

   Answer: b

   This patient's surgical intervention resulted in injury to the **inferior longitudinal fasciculus** (ILF), particularly the posterior fibers. This white matter tract is typically involved in a variety of brain functions, however; its posterior portion plays a major role in visual processing and visually associated behaviors (eg, reading). Therefore, ILF disruption in this patient would most likely lead to **alexia**. Other visual functions such as object and face recognition may also be impaired. Bilateral lesions are usually required for the full clinical picture as injury to one tract can be compensated for by the contralateral portion. Moreover, it has been shown that disturbances in ILF are the basis for visual hallucinations in some disorders (especially schizophrenia).

   Points to remember

   Inferior longitudinal fasciculus (ILF) can be injured during surgical resection of infiltrative brain tumors. This typically results in visually associated symptoms such as visual agnosia, prosopagnosia, and alexia.

6. A 54-year-old man is admitted to the hospital for evaluation of right-sided arm weakness and numbness over the past month. Brain MRI revealed a left frontoparietal lesion predominantly involving the postcentral gyrus. Glioblastoma is suspected and further evaluation is required. Which of the following is the most appropriate imaging modality for surgical planning in this patient?

   (a) Short Tau Inversion Recovery (STIR) imaging
   (b) Diffusion tensor (DT) imaging
   (c) CT scan of the head
   (d) Fluid-attenuated inversion recovery (FLAIR)
   (e) Functional MRI (fMRI)
   (f) High-definition fiber tractography (HDFT)

   Answer: e

   This patient right-sided upper extremity weakness along with numbness suggests the involvement of the precentral and postcentral gyrus. The corticospinal tract is typically responsible for controlling motor function and thus tumor displacement of this tract would most likely result in a weakness (as seen in this patient). Given the patient's age and gradual worsening of the symptoms, this most likely represents a growing neoplastic lesion (particularly malignant due to the rapid progression within 1 month).

Although the conventional white matter tractography, diffusion tensor imaging (DTI), is usually used for preoperative planning to maximize surgical resection while preserving adjacent tracts, some cases are quite complex due to the involvement of multiple crossing fibers. This issue has been resolved by using a more advanced imaging modality, the high-definition fiber tractography (HDFT), particularly in the setting of edematous zones surrounding high-grade cerebral neoplasms. The characterization of the fiber bundles provided by HDFT is superior to that of traditional DTI due to its ability to delineate the spatial relationship of white matter tracts in a 3D manner. Therefore, this allows the surgeon to accurately plan the optimal surgical approach and minimize otherwise unavoidable extensive resection.

Points to remember

For patients with infiltrative high-grade brain gliomas that involve multiple white matter tracts, a 3D characterization of the spatial anatomical orientation can be provided by high-definition fiber tractography.

7. A 65-year-old woman is brought to the office by her spouse due to cognitive impairment. The patient has been mildly forgetful over the past 4 months, with a further significant decline in the last 2 months. She performs most daily activities independently but must be reminded frequently to perform basic self-care. She has had no gait abnormalities, motor weakness, or other neurological deficits. She still enjoys spending time with family and friends. She was recently diagnosed with an advanced primary brain tumor for which she has received partial brain radiotherapy. Which of the following subcortical structures would be most susceptible to radiotherapy-induced damage?

(a) Basal ganglia
(b) Thalamus
(c) Fornix
(d) Internal capsule
(e) Optical radiation
(f) Inferior longitudinal fasciculus
(g) Superior longitudinal fasciculus

Answer: c

This patient's 4-month memory deficit in the setting of recent brain radiation is highly suggestive of **radiation-induced white matter damage.** White matter fibers that comprise the limbic system are the most susceptible white matter tracts to radiotherapy of the brain. Of these, fornix, cingulum, and corpus callosum are the most affected. This typically occurs in a dose-dependent fashion. Radiosensitivity of the limbic system and resultant dysfunction of cognitive abilities following radiotherapy indicates that these white matter fibers play a critical role in memory formation.

Points to remember

Fornix, cingulum bundles, and corpus callosum are the most susceptible white matter tracts to radiotherapy of the brain.

8. A 9-year-old boy is brought to the office by his parents due to worsening headaches over the past month. Gait is slow and unsteady. A brain MRI revealed a posterior fossa mass consistent with medulloblastoma. Surgical removal of the tumor was successfully performed without postoperative complications. A follow-up evaluation after 2 years revealed a generalized decrease in cognitive performance which was noted by his parents as deteriorating academic performance. A teacher has expressed concern that his grades have dropped from a B to a C average, that he is not engaged in class, and that his work has become "sloppy." Diffusion MRI demonstrated decreased fractional anisotropy (FA) associated with white matter volume loss. Which of the following is the most likely explanation of this patient current presentation?

  (a) Recurrence of medulloblastoma
  (b) Metastasis of medulloblastoma to supratentorial region
  (c) Microstructural damage to supratentorial frontal white matter
  (d) Hydrocephalus
  (e) Inadequate surgical removal of the tumor.

Answer: c

The 9-year-old child has undergone surgical removal of medulloblastoma and the subsequent cognitive decline and academic deterioration are suggestive of damage to **supratentorial frontal white matter fibers**. Survivors of medulloblastoma frequently have reduced white matter volume associated with neurocognitive dysfunction following surgery but prior to radiation and chemotherapy. The presentation may include a decline in working memory, intelligence, academic performance, and attention span (as seen in this patient). Diffusion-weighted magnetic resonance imaging (DWI) classically shows a decrease in fractional anisotropy (FA) which is most predominant in **corona radiata and corpus callosum**. This highlights the effect of surgical removal of posterior fossa tumors as well as the tumor itself on distant supratentorial white matter tracts, particularly frontal fibers.

Points to remember

Volume loss of supratentorial, frontal white matter fibers following surgical removal of posterior fossa tumors (eg, medulloblastoma) is responsible for the neurocognitive decline in survivors.

9. A 56-year-old man is being evaluated for a recent diagnosis of low-grade glioma. On neuroimaging, the tumor is found to be extending along the inferior fronto-occipital fasciculus (IFOF). The patient will most likely exhibit abnormality in which of the following high cortical functions?

(a) Spatial awareness
(b) Interpretation of sensory stimuli
(c) Executive functioning
(d) Semantic language
(e) Memory formation

Answer: d

The inferior fronto-occipital fasciculus (IFOF) is a long white matter tract that connects the occipital and frontal lobe on either side of the claustrum. It courses superficially to the temporal horn and laterally to the optic radiation before terminating variably at several areas of the cerebrum. Given this anatomical characterization, the IFOF plays a role in **semantic language** skills, especially naming. In addition, the tract links fibers from auditory and visual association cortices to the prefrontal area. This best explains the spread of disease between those areas, particularly the frontal and occipital lobes. It has been also implicated in the pathophysiology of Alzheimer disease, schizophrenia, and amnesia.

Points to remember

Dysfunction of inferior fronto-occipital fasciculus (IFOF) may lead to language disorders, especially semantic deficit. The spread of diseases along this tract can explain the spatial relationship between the area of deficit and the connected cortices.

10. A 58-year-old man is brought to the emergency department due to an episode of syncope, as stated by his wife who is a nurse practitioner. On physical examination, the patient is oriented to time, place, and person, but there is short-term memory impairment. Mild weakness of the left-sided extremities and a pronator drift of the left arm are present. Evidence of tongue biting is observed. An MRI of the brain shows a tumor involving the area anterior to the precentral gyrus in the right hemisphere. A brain biopsy revealed a malignant neoplasm and the patient was admitted to the hospital for surgical removal. The surgery was uncomplicated, and he is doing well. On postoperative day 4, the patient is found to be unable to move the left side of his body in addition to an inability to speak. Deep tendon reflexes are normal throughout. Which of the following is the most likely cause of this patient's current symptoms?

(a) Iatrogenic injury to the precentral gyrus
(b) Intracranial hemorrhage
(c) Postoperative stroke
(d) Supplementary motor area syndrome
(e) Inadequate removal of the tumor

Answer: d

This patient's left-sided hemiparesis with normal deep tendon reflexes following surgical removal of brain tumor involving supplementary motor area (SMA) is concerning for **SMA syndrome**. SMA is located anterior to the primary motor cortex (as seen in this patient). Importantly, the **frontal aslant tract** connects the precentral gyrus with the supplementary motor area. Damage to this fasciculus is thought to be responsible for the manifestations of SMA syndrome. These include transient loss of motor function usually on the contralateral side as well as mutism. Symptoms typically resolve completely within weeks to months. SMA syndrome most commonly results from neurosurgical resection of a tumor within this territory. Patients should be counseled about this syndrome and the transient nature of its symptoms.

Points to remember

The frontal aslant tract is a white matter tract that connects the primary motor cortex with the supplementary motor area. Neurosurgical resection of this tract can lead to SMA syndrome which typically presents as contralateral motor weakness and speech deficit.

11. A neurosurgery resident is looking at diffusion tensor (DT) tractography for a patient diagnosed with glioblastoma multiforme who is scheduled for surgery. The resident noticed a fiber tract extending from the anterior temporal lobe to the inferior frontal and orbital gyri. Which of the following white matter tracts is the resident currently observing?

    (a) Middle longitudinal fasciculus
    (b) Uncinate fasciculus (of Russell)
    (c) Inferior longitudinal fasciculus
    (d) Superior longitudinal fasciculus
    (e) Arcuate fasciculus
    (f) Cingulum

    Answer: b

    Uncinate fasciculus (of Russell) is a group of white matter association fibers that connects the anterior temporal lobe (particularly anterior parahippocampus and amygdala) with the inferior frontal and orbital gyri (ie. Orbitofrontal cortex). It is the last white matter tract to complete development in the human brain. The fibers course above the M1 segment of the middle cerebral artery in the anterior portion of the tract. Due to its anatomical distribution between the limbic system and orbitofrontal cortex, it is thought that damage to this tract is responsible for severe retrograde memory loss, especially following a trauma. Moreover, learning of associations through a trial and error method is strongly related to the microstructure of uncinate fasciculus.

    Points to remember

    Uncinate fasciculus (of Russel) is an association white matter tract that links the temporal lobe to the frontal lobe. It plays a crucial role in the maintenance of retrograde memory.

12. A 62-year-old woman with high-grade glioma is scheduled for surgery. Preoperative MRI reveals an infiltrative hyperintense lesion located deep to the corpus callosum and runs parallel to the superior longitudinal fasciculus posteriorly along the dorsal border of the caudate nucleus. Which of the following is most likely to appear in this patient after resection of this tumor?

    (a) Visual impairment
    (b) Auditory deficit
    (c) Language deficit
    (d) Impaired dexterity
    (e) Executive dysfunction
    (f) Impaired spatial awareness

    Answer: f

    This patient's tumor extension along the dorsal border of the caudate nucleus posteriorly, and its proximity to the superior longitudinal fasciculus is most likely involving the **superior occipitofrontal fasciculus** (SOFF). This white matter association tract connects the frontal and parietal lobes. It runs deep to the corpus callosum and then courses posteriorly adjacent to the dorsal border of the caudate nucleus and medial to superior longitudinal fasciculus, particularly the second branch (SLF II). The anterior portion of SOFF lies within the anterior limb of the internal capsule before terminating at the frontal lobe. Injury to this tract results in abnormal **spatial contextual awareness.** It is important to note that the nomenclature of this tract is relatively confusing as these fibers do not involve the occipital lobe.

    Points to remember

    The superior occipitofrontal fasciculus (SOFF) lies medial to the second branch of the superior longitudinal fasciculus SLF and is responsible for spatial awareness.

13. A 12-year-old boy is brought to the emergency department by his parents due to frequent staring episodes. The parents report that the patient's head usually tilts to the left, followed by left arm arbitrary movements during these episodes. The patient then begins swallowing and chewing his lips and rubbing his fingers. Each episode lasts 2–3 min and the patient appears lethargic and confused afterward. He had no incontinence during the event but was unable to move his right arm for 5–10 min afterward. The patient has no other medical conditions or allergies. He was previously doing well in school, but his grades have declined over the past few months, and his teacher has noted that he seems intermittently distracted. Vital signs are normal. The neurological exam is unremarkable. MRI of the brain showed diffuse hyperintensity involving white matter fibers located in angular, supramarginal, precentral, and postcentral gyri and terminating at the middle frontal gyrus. Which of the following is the most likely affected white matter tract?

    (a) Inferior longitudinal fasciculus
    (b) Middle longitudinal fasciculus

(c) Superior longitudinal fasciculus (branch II)
(d) Superior longitudinal fasciculus (branch III)
(e) Arcuate fasciculus
(f) Uncinate fasciculus

Answer: c

This patient likely had a focal seizure, defined as a seizure originating from a single hemisphere. Focal seizures can also spread to involve both cerebral hemispheres and cause impaired awareness, as seen with this patient's subsequent staring episode. This patient's clinical presentation indicates a structural lesion that triggered his seizure episodes. The MRI of the brain showed a hyperintense lesion most likely involving the **superior longitudinal fasciculus (branch II)** which normally connects the prefrontal cortex with the inferior parietal cortex. The tract courses through the following gyri: angular, supramarginal, pre- and post-central, and middle frontal gyri. Because of the involvement of the parietal lobe (generally responsible for the interpretation of sensory stimuli) and parts of the temporal lobe (partly responsible for memory formation), these fibers are typically involved in abnormalities of **spatial working memory** needed for orientation in space and navigation around familiar environments.

Points to remember

Damage to the superior longitudinal fasciculus (branch II) can lead to disorders of spatial memory.

14. A 73-year-old male comes to the emergency department due to a sudden onset of confusion, ataxia, nausea, and disorientation. The patient was recently diagnosed with systemic melanoma that is controlled with a nivolumab regimen. An initial computed tomography (CT) scan revealed an area of left hypodensity measuring 3×4 cm adjacent to and compressing a fiber tract that courses caudally on the roof and lateral wall of the temporal horn of the ventricular system, along with other multiple lesions throughout the brain. Surgical removal of this lesion will most likely decompress which of the following tracts in this patient?

(a) Auditory tract
(b) Middle longitudinal fasciculus
(c) Inferior longitudinal fasciculus
(d) Optic radiation
(e) Fornix
(f) Corona radiata

Answer: d

This patient's history of systemic melanoma suggests a distant spread to the brain. Metastatic disease of the CNS is the most common cause of brain tumors. The hypodense lesion seen in this patient is consistent with a metastatic melanoma lesion. The superior and lateral anatomical location around the temporal horn of the ventricular system most likely involves the **optic radiation** which typically originates from the lateral geniculate bodies bilaterally. This white matter tract is composed of three major bundles: posterior, central, and anterior bundles. The latter is also known as "Meyer's loop" due to its curved nature around the tip of the temporal horn. This patient's metastatic lesion has compressed Meyer's loop of the optic radiation. Superior quadrantanopia is also expected to be found in this patient as Meyer's loop receives optic information from the inferior lateral part of the retina.

Points to remember

Optic radiation projects from the lateral geniculate body. Its anterior bundle "Meyer's loop" courses on the roof and around the tip of the temporal horn.

15. A researcher is studying the anatomical characterization of the various white matter tracts in the human brain. She learned that the superior longitudinal fasciculus (SLF) is composed of three major bundles. Damage in which of the following branches of SLF is most likely to result in aphasia?

    (a) SLF (branch I)
    (b) SLF (branch II)
    (c) SLF (branch III)
    (d) Temporo-parietal branch of SLF (SLF-tp)

    Answer: d

    The superior longitudinal fasciculus is an association white matter tract that connects the four lobes of the brain. Although there is no clear consensus on the subcomponents of this tract, it has been shown that there are several major branches that are consistently seen in diffusion tensor (DT) imaging. These are the SLF branches I, II, III, and the temporoparietal branch (SLF-tp). The SLF-tp. As the name implies, this branch connects the temporal lobe with the parietal lobe and is thought to participate in language processing, especially interpretation. Therefore, a lesion in this branch would typically result in receptive or "fluent" aphasia due to the proximity of these fibers from Wernicke's area.

    Points to remember

    There are several major branches of the superior longitudinal fasciculus: SLF I, II, III, and tp. The SLF-tp bundle is language-related and injury to this area results in aphasia.

16. During the dissection of a human brain for teaching purposes, an anatomist found two semi-parallel bundles of white matter running immediately below the splenium of the corpus callosum. Rostrally, they form the anterior wall of the lateral ventricle before they course superomedially to the thalamus. Which of the following structures represent the origin and terminal destination of these fibers, respectively?

    (a) Thalamus, hippocampus
    (b) Cingulum, pineal gland
    (c) Mamillary body, supraoptic nucleus
    (d) Tectum, hypothalamus
    (e) Hippocampus, mamillary bodies

    Answer: e

The observed white matter tract most likely represents the **fornix**, which is comprised of two thick bundles inferior to the corpus callosum. The fornix initially **originates** as a thin, efferent group of fibers **from the hippocampus**. These fibers thicken to form the crura of the fornix bilaterally prior to being connected by the hippocampal commissure. The crura then fuse anterior to the splenium of the corpus callosum into the body of fornix, passing freely in the inferior border of the septum pellucidum. At this level, the fornix aligns with the foremen of Monro and forms the anterior wall of the lateral ventricle. It then bifurcates into the columns of the fornix before joining the **mammillary bodies** on each side. The mammillothalamic tract continues from the mamillary bodies to the anterior nucleus of the thalamus.

Points to remember

The fornix originates in the hippocampus, runs inferiorly to the corpus callosum, and then terminates at the mamillary bodies.

17. A 32-year-old, left-handed, African American woman comes to the emergency room due to confusion and severe headaches. Her husband noted that the patient was running into furniture lately, especially on the right side. He also reports that his wife was weak on her right side where she has been dropping objects. MRI of the brain was immediately obtained revealing a large left-sided temporal-parietal-occipital lesion with heterogenous enhancement and extensive adjacent edema. After stabilization, the patient was counseled on the available management plans, including surgical intervention. The neurosurgeon explained the benefits and adverse effects of the surgery as well as alternative treatments. The patient agreed to surgical removal of the lesion and emphasized the importance of preserving her language function as she works as a motivational speaker in a well-known international company. Which of the following is the most appropriate intraoperative technique for this patient?

(a) Craniotomy with transcranial motor mapping
(b) Awake craniotomy with direct electrical stimulation
(c) Awake craniotomy without electrical stimulation
(d) Craniotomy under general anesthesia with intraoperative navigation based on preoperative MRI
(e) Craniotomy under general anesthesia with intraoperative fluorescence imaging

Answer: b

This young patient has subacute nature of symptom progression. Given her symptoms and MRI characteristics, this patient most likely has high-grade glioma**.** In order to achieve safe, maximal resection while preserving the language area (due to the eloquent location of the tumor, right side in this patient), continuous intraoperative monitoring is required. This is typically achieved by performing the surgery in an **awake** manner with **direct electrical stimulation and intraoperative navigation**. Therefore, this patient requires left-sided, awake craniotomy for tumor resection with cortical and subcortical direct electrical stimulation and mapping, particularly for language function. Intraoperative brain mapping can be also used for preserving other brain areas such as those involved in sensorimotor, visual, spatial, and cognitive functions.

Points to remember

Awake craniotomy with direct electrical stimulation and intraoperative navigation can be used for functional mapping and maximizing the resection of infiltrative lesions within or surrounding the language region in the eloquent cortex.

18. A 36-year-old male presented to the clinic secondary to dull aching headaches involving the right side of the skull and spreading toward the posterior left side occasionally. MRI of the brain revealed a homogenous FLAIR hyperintense lesion located in the right insula. An intraoperative awake mapping with cortical and subcortical electrostimulation is recommended to preserve the language region. To avoid provoking seizures while providing sufficient stimulation, which of the following pairs of stimulation frequency and current form should be maintained during the electrostimulation and intraoperative mapping?

   (a) 20 Hz, 18 mA
   (b) 10 Hz, 25 mA
   (c) 2 Hz, 4 mA
   (d) 55 Hz, 6 mA
   (e) 80 Hz, 20 mA

   Answer: d

   This young patient likely has low-grade glioma in the right insular lobe. Operative resection was recommended due to symptoms, the accessible location of the tumor, and the patient's age. Surgical removal for this patient's tumor typically requires an intraoperative mapping with cortical and subcortical direct electrostimulation to maximize resection. Safety and sufficient stimulation should be taken into consideration simultaneously when performing brain functional mapping. Consequently, the probe electrode should be set on alternating monopolar square wave pulses (1 ms), low-frequency range of (50–60 Hz), a stimulus duration of 3–5 s, and slowly increasing the current power up to 8 mA. Of the given choices, choice (D) with 55 Hz, 6 mA is considered safe and sufficient. The subdural electrode measures are similar to the probe electrode except that the power of current can be increased up to 15 mA. Importantly, post-stimulation discharges, represented by false positive responses, should be carefully monitored and suppressed by icy ringer solution and propofol at all times during the mapping.

   Points to remember

   Care should be taken to avoid provoking seizures during awake craniotomy with brain mapping when using the electrodes during stimulation. An acceptable safe range of frequency and current power is 50–60 Hz and 2–8 mA (probe electrode), 2–15 (subdural electrode).

19. During awake craniotomy for removal of low-grade glioma in the left insular lobe, an electrostimulation with cortical and subcortical mapping was performed. After sensorimotor mapping, the neurosurgeon attempted to preserve language function due to the involvement of the dominant insula using subcortical language mapping. Which of the following white matter tracts most likely runs through the insula and hence must be preserved when possible?

(a) Inferior fronto-occipital tract
(b) Middle longitudinal fasciculus
(c) Arcuate fasciculus
(d) Superior longitudinal tract
(e) Inferior longitudinal tract

Answer: a

Language processing is typically carried out through dorsal and ventral pathways. The dorsal pathway deals with the integration of auditory and motor functions for optimal articulation. In contrast, the ventral pathway matches sounds and their meaning in the brain. Notably, the ventral pathway with its two major tracts; **uncinate fasciculus** and **inferior fronto-occipital fasciculus** pass through the insula. To benefit from continuous monitoring during the assessment of real-time language function in generally anesthetized patients, awake craniotomy with subcortical mapping is usually required. Therefore, subcortical language mapping is of paramount importance during the resection of tumors within the dominant insula.

Points to remember

Subcortical language mapping during awake craniotomy for insular lesions is important to preserve language function.

20. A 55-year-old male presented with right-sided upper extremity weakness and numbness over the past several weeks. The patient says, "I think it all began last month when my wife and I started to fight more than usual". The symptoms became more severe today. He has a history of hypercholesterolemia and hypertension. He has no known psychiatric history. Due to the subacute nature of his symptoms, his primary physician ordered a brain MRI which revealed left-sided hyperintense, ill-defined frontoparietal lesion with extensions to the region adjacent to the frontal operculum and external to the claustrum with no contrast enhancement. The decision was made to undergo awake surgical resection using intraoperative brain mapping with direct electrical stimulation. Based on the tumor location, which of the following tasks should be assessed intraoperatively while mapping the frontal operculum and adjacent temporal lobe?

(a) Continuous movement with his hands
(b) Disturbance of tongue movement after stimulation of the corresponding area
(c) Visual acuity
(d) Automated speech and object naming
(e) Sensory function

Answer: d

The clinical presentation and brain MRI of this patient are suggestive of a low-grade glioma. Several studies have shown overall prolonged survival with early maximal resection. Optimization of surgical removal is key to the successful management of these tumors as well as better survival rates. For this purpose, intraoperative navigation with direct electrical stimulation for functional brain mapping is usually indicated. In this patient, the tumor is located in the proximity of the frontal operculum and the superior portion of the temporal lobe, a region occupied by the inferior fronto-occipital fasciculus (IFOF). This white matter tract is heavily involved in language processing, particularly semantic language, and naming. As a result, tasks such as automated speech (eg, counting, reciting days of the week), and object naming (eg, in response to pictures) during the surgery are used to map language, preserving perilesional white matter tracts responsible for language production and processing.

Points to remember

Task such as object naming is typically used to map language areas during awake surgical removal of tumors that are located in the eloquent cortex and adjacent to main language bundles.

21. A previously healthy, 44-year-old farmer is brought to the emergency department due to new-onset confusion and generalized tonic-clonic seizures. In the emergency department, blood pressure is 174/130 mm Hg, the pulse is 98/min, and the pulse oximetry is 98% on 100% FiO_2. On examination, he is found to have weakness in his right extremities, more pronounced in his upper arms. Non-contrast CT scan of the head demonstrated a left frontoparietal hypodense lesion with extensive surrounding edema. MRI of the brain was then ordered which confirmed the physician's suspicion of malignant neoplasm, likely glioblastoma multiforme. Following stabilization, the patient was counseled about the risks and benefits of surgery as well as the prognosis. Which of the following factors is significantly implicated in the assessment of this patient's prognosis?

(a) Gender
(b) Concomitant comorbidities and family history
(c) Migration along white matter tracts
(d) Time from symptoms to diagnosis
(e) Degree of adjacent edema

Answer: c

This patient has glioblastoma multiforme (GBM), one of the most aggressive primary brain tumors in adults. The prognosis is still dismal despite the current advancements in medical and surgical therapies. Survival can be moderately predicted by several factors including but not exclusive to age, postoperative residual tumor, and adjuvant therapy. **GBM** is notorious for infiltrating and migrating along subcortical white matter tracts. GBMs that **intersect white matter tract**s like inferior fronto-occipital fasciculus, and inferior longitudinal fasciculus (ILF), tend to have a poor prognosis regardless of any therapy. This is attributed to the ability of the tumor to reach vital areas, especially in the brainstem, responsible for cardiopulmonary function (eg, breathing and hemodynamic stability). Interestingly, involvement of left ILF has been associated with decreased progressing-free survival but not overall survival. This indicates that white matter tract infiltration plays a key role in predicting prognosis in patients with GBM.

Points to remember

Intersection and migration of malignant gliomas along white matter tracts may correlate with poor prognosis.

22. A 35-year-old musician is undergoing awake operative removal for low-grade glioma in a functional area. The neurosurgeon is utilizing intraoperative navigation with direct electrical stimulation to minimize postoperative functional deficits. During subcortical stimulation of the perilesional region, specifically inferior and lateral to the temporal horn and under the optic pathways, the patient exhibited disturbances in spontaneous speech and picture naming. Which of the following fiber tracts was the neurosurgeon specifically targeting?

    (a) Superior longitudinal fasciculus
    (b) Middle longitudinal fasciculus
    (c) Inferior longitudinal fasciculus
    (d) Inferior fronto-occipital fasciculus
    (e) Optic radiation
    (f) Uncinate fasciculus
    (g) Arcuate fasciculus

    Answer: c

    This patient's intraoperative speech difficulties following direct electrical stimulation are consistent with targeting the **inferior longitudinal fasciculus (ILF)**. ILF is a long association white matter tract that connects the occipital lobe with the anterior portion of the temporal lobe. It lies in close contact with the lateral wall of the temporal horn at the level of the inferior temporal gyrus and courses beneath the optic radiation. ILF has been strongly associated with language function, especially visual processing of written language and language comprehension. The surgeon targeted the ILF in this patient which explains the language abnormalities during electrical stimulation.

    Points to remember

    The inferior longitudinal fasciculus runs near the temporal horn in the superior temporal gyrus. Intraoperative stimulation of this fiber tract may result in speech disturbances and semantic deficits.

23. A neurosurgery resident is assisting with a sleep-awake-sleep operative removal of high-grade glioma in a 43-year-old male patient, using brain mapping and electrical stimulation. While approaching the lesion through the transsylvian route, the attendant surgeon asked the resident about an important landmark to

help localize the inferior longitudinal fasciculus and inferior occipitofrontal fasciculus. Which of the following anatomical landmarks was the attendant questioning the resident about?

(a) Frontal horns of lateral ventricles
(b) Sylvian fissure
(c) Middle cerebral artery
(d) Lenticulostriate artery
(e) Roof of temporal horn
(f) Central sulcus

Answer: e

Inferior longitudinal fasciculus (ILF) and inferior occipitofrontal fasciculus (IFOF) are both white matter association tracts that run in close proximity to each other. An important anatomical landmark that facilitates distinguishing the two tracts is the **roof of the temporal horn of lateral ventricles**. This landmark is bounded inferiorly by ILF and superiorly by IFOF. It is also important to note that ILF courses laterally and inferiorly to optic pathways. IFOF, on the other hand, runs superiorly and medially to optic radiations.

Points to remember

The roof of the temporal horn is a useful anatomical landmark in localizing the inferior longitudinal fasciculus (ILF) and inferior occipitofrontal fasciculus (IFOF). ILF runs inferior to the temporal horn whereas IFOF runs superior to it.

24. A 75-year-old, left-handed woman is brought to the emergency department by her daughter for behavioral issues. Her daughter explains that she has "not been herself" since visiting her a few months ago. The patient has become increasingly irritable with her daughter for no clear reason. The daughter says, "my mom inconsistently has had difficulties differentiating between sounds during the same period. Yesterday, she complained of hearing the sound of a plane taking off when I was using the microwave". MRI of the brain was obtained and revealed a hyperintense lesion involving the right superior temporal lobe in addition to a low T1 signal involving the left temporal lobe, indicating previous ischemic stroke. On brainstem auditory evoked response (BAER), long-latency responses (LLR), and middle latency responses (MLR) are completely abolished. The physician suspects malignant lesions affecting a major white matter tract. Which of the following structures are anatomically connected via the most likely involved fiber tract?

(a) Cingulum and anterior thalamus
(b) Lateral geniculate body and occipital lobe
(c) Right and left hemisphere
(d) Orbital cortices and hippocampus
(e) Anterior thalamus and hippocampus
(f) Medial geniculate body and Broadman area 41/42

Answer: f

This patient's difficulties differentiating environmental sounds and bilateral involvement of temporal lobes on MRI is consistent with **cortical deafness**, a rare form of sensorineural hearing loss. Although the anatomy of the ear is normal, patients are typically unaware of the sounds (inability to process auditory information). This is usually the result of bilateral damage to the primary auditory cortex in the superior temporal lobes, as seen in this patient. The auditory pathway (acoustic radiation) is comprised of heavily myelinated fibers that run from the **medial geniculate body** of the thalamus toward the **primary auditory cortex** (Broadman are 41 and 42).

Points to remember

Bilateral damage to acoustic radiation results in a rare form of sensorineural hearing loss, cortical (cerebral) deafness. Patients typically present with an inability to interpret environmental sounds manifested as deafness despite normal peripheral auditory structures.

25. A 32-year-old, previously healthy woman comes to the office due to worsening symptoms of menstrual irregularities. Five months ago, the patient began missing menstrual periods irregularly. A trial of progesterone failed to improve the patient's symptoms. She reports that she has been walking into objects over the same duration. This morning, the patient developed a double vision that spontaneously resolved within minutes. An initial CT scan of the head demonstrated a large 3 × 2.4 × 2.2 cm suprasellar lesion with a displacement of the optic chiasm. A staged endonasal and transcranial resection was recommended. During the surgery, the surgeon pointed at a structure crossing the midline immediately above the optic tracts. Which of the following represents the most likely structure being addressed here?

   (a) Optic nerve
   (b) Anterior cerebral artery
   (c) Anterior commissure
   (d) Anterior communicating artery
   (e) Preoptic nucleus

   Answer: c

   Anterior commissure represents an interhemispheric white matter tract that crosses the midline immediately **superior** to the **optic tracts** and **inferior** to the **rostrum** of the corpus callosum. At the midline, it begins as a compact bundle of fibers below the globus pallidus and within the caudate nucleus; then it fans out into the temporal and orbitofrontal cortex on each side. It lies anterior to the columns of the fornix and contains decussating fibers from olfactory tracts. Additionally, the anterior commissure serves to connect the amygdalae bilaterally. The majority of fibers composing this tract merge lateroposteriorly with the inferior fronto-occipital fasciculus, with some fibers joining the uncinate fasciculus. It is thought that anterior commissure contributes to a variety of brain functions, especially pain perception olfaction, and sexual function.

Points to remember

The anterior commissure is one of the interhemispheric white matter tracts and is located superiorly to the optic tracts and inferior to the rostrum of the corpus callosum across the midline.

26. A diffusion tensor imaging (DTI) of a 55-year-old male with low-grade glioma shows an involvement of a distinct white matter tract extending from the poles of temporal lobes, coursing through the substance of the superior temporal gyrus toward the inferior part of the parietal lobe around the angular gyrus. Which of the following represents the structure being described in this patient?

    (a) Superior longitudinal fasciculus
    (b) Middle longitudinal fasciculus
    (c) Inferior longitudinal fasciculus
    (d) Inferior occipito-frontal fasciculus
    (e) Uncincate fasciculus

    Answer: b

    The first description of **middle longitudinal fasciculus (MLF)** was in monkeys. It has been shown that this white matter tract that connects the inferior parietal lobules with the superior temporal gyri bilaterally. This was then confirmed in human brains via modern imaging techniques such as diffusion tensor imaging (DTI). MLF contributes to language function through participation in both the ventral and dorsal routes responsible for language processing. However, this fascicle may not be essential to the processing of language as removal of this fiber bundle or intraoperative electrostimulation have not been associated with postoperative language deficit or abnormalities in picture naming, respectively. MLF fibers run parallel to the extreme capsule and may extend to occipital lobes posteriorly. The function of this bundle is still not established despite the anatomical relation to language tracts.

    Points to remember

    Tumor involvement of the middle longitudinal fasciculus (MLF) may not lead to an apparent language deficit as this white matter tract is not essential for language processing.

27. A 59-year-old man is brought to the office by his wife due to personality changes. She says, "he began behaving strangely over the past 4 months and became very irritable and agitated almost all the time. He recently lost his job due to involvement in an altercation with his coworker which he used to like ever since he began this job." On neurological examination, mild weakness in the right lower extremity is noted. The patient reports that he has had syncopal episodes during the same period. MRI of the brain was ordered and revealed a parieto-occipital homogenous signal on T1 and T2 images with distinct borders just above the corpus callosum. A brain biopsy confirmed the diagnosis of grade-2 oligodendroglioma. Diffusion tensor imaging (DTI) was obtained for presurgical planning. The images show the involvement of a collection of fibers extending from the area above the corpus callosum toward the entorhinal cor-

tex. Which of the following white matter bundles is most likely to be affected in this patient?

(a) Subcallosal fasciculus
(b) Superior longitudinal fasciculus
(c) Arcuate fasciculus
(d) Cingulum
(e) Uncinate fasciculus

Answer: d

This patient has seizures, lower extremity weakness, and personality changes which along with radiographical characteristics on MRI and the subacute nature of symptoms are consistent with a malignant brain neoplasm. This was confirmed through a biopsy which showed low-grade (2) oligodendroglioma. According to the updated WHO classification of CNS tumors, diagnosis of oligodendroglioma is made by identifying an infiltrative glioma with IDH mutation and 1p19q codeletion. In this patient, the tumor has infiltrated the **cingulum**, as seen in DT imaging. The cingulum is a collection of white matter fibers located centrally right above the corpus callosum. It terminates at the entorhinal cortices bilaterally and plays a role in emotion, pain, and memory (limbic system). It has been also shown that fibers frequently exiting and entering the cingulum contribute to the connection of parietal, frontal, and temporal lobes in both hemispheres. Because of this parallel fashion of fibers arrangement, lesion to the cingulum results only in mild neurological deficits.

Points to remember

The cingulum extends from the cingulate gyrus right above the corpus callosum to the entorhinal cortices. It is involved in pain, emotion, and memory formation, among other limbic system functions.

28. According to the recent model for language processing, it has been suggested that the dual stream model is composed of two main pathways: the dorsal and ventral routes. The dorsal route was found to be formed from the fibers of the arcuate fasciculus (AF) and the third subcomponent of the superior longitudinal fasciculus (SLFIII). A diffusion tensor imaging (DTI) of a 77-year-old-man shows disruption of the dorsal stream integrity due to metastatic lesions and resultant adjacent edema. Which of the following speech functions is primarily affected in this patient?

(a) Sensory-motor integration
(b) Mapping sound to meaning
(c) Auditory perception
(d) Visual-auditory integration
(e) Vocabulary access

Answer: a

This patient's DTI shows metastatic lesions along the **dorsal stream** of speech pathway, which is mainly involved in mapping auditory afferent information to motor speech functions (ie **sensory-motor integration**). The recent model of language processing is typically subdivided into two major routes: the dorsal and ventral streams. The uncinate fasciculus (UF) and third branch of superior longitudinal fasciculus (SLF-III) form the dorsal pathway, whereas the ventral stream is comprised of the inferior longitudinal fasciculus (ILF), the UF, and the inferior fronto-occipital fasciculus (IFOF). The latter is responsible for semantic language and language comprehension (ie integration of auditory stimuli to sound meanings) via connecting the middle temporal lobe with the prefrontal area. On the other hand, the dorsal pathway connects the superior temporal lobes with the frontal area, specifically the premotor cortices. Of note, the middle longitudinal fasciculus is involved in both streams.

Points to remember

The language function can be categorized anatomically into ventral and dorsal streams. The dorsal stream is responsible for sensory-motor integration whereas the ventral route contributes to auditory comprehension of language.

29. A 64-year-old woman was referred for evaluation of right-sided hemiparesis and aphasia. She has daily temporal headaches and feels quite fatigued. The patient used to smoke cigarettes but now uses vaporized nicotine. Her medical history is unremarkable. Temperature is 36.6 °C (97.8 F), blood pressure is 128/74 mm Hg, and pulse is 88/min. She is well-appearing. There are sensory deficits in her feet, but her reflexes and strength are mildly diminished. Brain MRI shows a large left frontoparietal mass. Diffusion tensor (DT) imaging shows displacement of the fibers connecting the thalamus and cerebral cortex. Which of the following functions is primarily supported by the affected white matter tract in this patient?

(a) Emotion and memory formation
(b) Control of appetite
(c) Regulation of internal body temperature
(d) Relay of sensory and motor information
(e) Spatial awareness

Answer: d

This patient has headaches, fatigue, hemiparesis, and aphasia. In combination with the left frontoparietal mass, this is most likely suggestive of a malignant lesion compressing the motor strip. The DT calculation shows displacement of **thalamocortical radiation,** a critical white matter tract with reciprocal connections that is larger and more complex in humans than in other mammals. These fibers pass through the internal capsule, particularly the anterior and retrolenticular segments. Its superior extension represents the corona radiata before terminating widely at the cerebral cortex (layer IV). Of the functions mentioned above, **relaying sensory and motor information** to the post- and pre-central gyrus, respectively, is the most likely correct answer. Other functions include carrying visual and auditory input through the lateral and medial geniculate nuclei.

Points to remember

Thalamic radiation is a white matter fiber tract that receives major sensory and motor inputs and relays it to appropriate cortical connections for processing and integration.

30. A 22-year-old male presented to the emergency department with severe nausea, vomiting, tinnitus, and frontal headaches. The headaches worsen with bending forward and are simultaneously associated with double vision. Recently, he fell while getting up at night to use the bathroom. Vital signs are normal without orthostasis. On examination, he has difficulty getting up from a chair. BMI is 22 kg/m^2. An emergent non-contrast CT scan of the head demonstrated an exophytic brainstem tumor arising from the fourth ventricle with a vague area of distorted architecture surrounding the tumor. A diagnosis of pilocytic astrocytoma was suspected. MRI of the spine and brain could not distinguish the semi-infiltrative region seen in CT from vasogenic edema. Which of the following imaging techniques allows for determining whether the patient is a good candidate for surgery?

   (a) Functional MRI
   (b) PET scan
   (c) Contrast CT scan of the head
   (d) MRA
   (e) Fluid-attenuated inversion recovery (FLAIR)
   (f) Short Tau Inversion Recovery (STIR) imaging
   (g) Diffusion Tensor Imaging (DTI)

   Answer: g

   This patient with nausea, vomiting, headaches, tinnitus, visual changes, dizziness (falling down while getting up), and evidence of mass in the fourth ventricle on the CT scan has an exophytic cervicomedullary junction tumor. These tumors typically extend rostrally and caudally into the medulla and cervical spinal cord, respectively. The neurosurgeon should weigh the benefits of surgical removal against resultant morbidity. Therefore, the decision on whether to perform surgery depends on the radiographic appearance of the MRI (CT is not reliable due to bone artifact at the level of the foramen magnum). Surgery is recommended when low-grade tumors are suspected and improvement in neurological deficits can be achieved with total or maximal resection. When the conventional imaging techniques cannot characterize a low-grade and local tumor, surgery is deferred until more accurate anatomical delineation can be obtained, as the resultant morbidity from debulking an otherwise high-grade invasive tumor will be detrimental to the patient. For this purpose, conventional imaging combined with **diffusion tensor imaging** (DTI) can differentiate between white matter tract infiltration and displacement in this highly compacted region of the spinal cord. Observation of normal anatomical integrity of these white matter tracts (by the ability to trace tracts in relation to an adjacent tumor with no direct infiltration) indicates low-grade tumors, and that the patient is a good candidate for surgical removal.

Points to remember

Diffusion tensor imaging (DTI) is critical to determine resectability of cervicomedullary junction tumors.

Test your learning and check your understanding of this book's contents: use the "Springer Nature Flashcards" app to access questions using https://sn.pub/3HwHCw To use the app, please follow the instructions in Chap. 1.

Bibliography

1. Voets NL, Bartsch A, Plaha P. Brain white matter fibre tracts: a review of functional neuro-oncological relevance. J Neurol Neurosurg Psychiatry. 2017;88(12):1017–25.
2. Witwer BP, Moftakhar R, Hasan KM, Deshmukh P, Haughton V, Field A, Arfanakis K, Noyes J, Moritz CH, Meyerand ME, Rowley HA. Diffusion-tensor imaging of white matter tracts in patients with cerebral neoplasm. J Neurosurg. 2002;97(3):568–75.
3. Bourekas EC, Varakis K, Bruns D, Christoforidis GA, Baujan M, Slone HW, Kehagias D. Lesions of the corpus callosum: MR imaging and differential considerations in adults and children. Am J Roentgenol. 2002;179(1):251–7.
4. Wycoco V, Shroff M, Sudhakar S, Lee W. White matter anatomy: what the radiologist needs to know. Neuroimaging Clin. 2013;23(2):197–216.
5. Herbet G, Zemmoura I, Duffau H. Functional anatomy of the inferior longitudinal fasciculus: from historical reports to current hypotheses. Front Neuroanat. 2018;12:77.
6. Abhinav K, Yeh FC, Mansouri A, Zadeh G, Fernandez-Miranda JC. High-definition fiber tractography for the evaluation of perilesional white matter tracts in high-grade glioma surgery. Neuro-Oncology. 2015;17(9):1199–209.
7. Connor M, Karunamuni R, McDonald C, Seibert T, White N, Moiseenko V, Bartsch H, Farid N, Kuperman J, Krishnan A, Dale A. Regional susceptibility to dose-dependent white matter damage after brain radiotherapy. Radiother Oncol. 2017;123(2):209–17.
8. Glass JO, Ogg RJ, Hyun JW, Harreld JH, Schreiber JE, Palmer SL, Li Y, Gajjar AJ, Reddick WE. Disrupted development and integrity of frontal white matter in patients treated for pediatric medulloblastoma. Neuro-Oncology. 2017;19(10):1408–18.
9. Conner AK, Briggs RG, Sali G, Rahimi M, Baker CM, Burks JD, Glenn CA, Battiste JD, Sughrue ME. A connectomic atlas of the human cerebrum—chapter 13: tractographic description of the inferior fronto-occipital fasciculus. Operat Neurosurg. 2018;15(Suppl 1):S436–43.
10. Mandonnet E, Capelle L, Duffau H. Extension of paralimbic low grade gliomas: toward an anatomical classification based on white matter invasion patterns. J Neuro-Oncol. 2006;78(2):179–85.
11. Potgieser AR, De Jong BM, Wagemakers M, Hoving EW, Groen RJ. Insights from the supplementary motor area syndrome in balancing movement initiation and inhibition. Front Hum Neurosci. 2014;28(8):960.
12. Metoki A, Alm KH, Wang Y, Ngo CT, Olson IR. Never forget a name: white matter connectivity predicts person memory. Brain Struct Funct. 2017;222(9):4187–201.
13. Liang W, Yu Q, Wang W, Dhollander T, Suluba E, Li Z, Xu F, Hu Y, Tang Y, Liu S. Subdivision of superior longitudinal fasciculus in human neonatal brain. Res Square. 2017.
14. Wang X, Pathak S, Stefaneanu L, Yeh FC, Li S, Fernandez-Miranda JC. Subcomponents and connectivity of the superior longitudinal fasciculus in the human brain. Brain Struct Funct. 2016;221(4):2075–92.

15. Bernal B, Altman N. The connectivity of the superior longitudinal fasciculus: a tractography DTI study. Magn Reson Imaging. 2010;28(2):217–25.
16. Lövblad KO, Schaller K, Vargas MI. The fornix and limbic system. InSeminars in ultrasound, CT and MRI. WB Saunders. 2014;35(5):459–73.
17. Pallud J, Rigaux-Viode O, Corns R, Muto J, Lopez CL, Mellerio C, Sauvageon X, Dezamis E. Direct electrical bipolar electrostimulation for functional cortical and subcortical cerebral mapping in awake craniotomy. Practical considerations. Neurochirurgie. 2017;63(3):164–74.
18. Mikuni N, Miyamoto S. Surgical treatment for glioma: extent of resection applying functional neurosurgery. Neurol Med Chir. 2010;50(9):720–6.
19. Yamao Y, Matsumoto R, Kikuchi T, Yoshida K, Kunieda T, Miyamoto S. Intraoperative brain mapping by cortico-cortical evoked potential. Front Hum Neurosci. 2021;18(15):55.
20. Jakola AS, Myrmel KS, Kloster R, Torp SH, Lindal S, Unsgård G, Solheim O. Comparison of a strategy favoring early surgical resection vs a strategy favoring watchful waiting in low-grade gliomas. JAMA. 2012;308(18):1881–8.
21. Rofes A, Miceli G. Language mapping with verbs and sentences in awake surgery: a review. Neuropsychol Rev. 2014;24(2):185–99.
22. Mickevicius NJ, Carle AB, Bluemel T, Santarriaga S, Schloemer F, Shumate D, Connelly J, Schmainda KM, LaViolette PS. Location of brain tumor intersecting white matter tracts predicts patient prognosis. J Neuro-Oncol. 2015;125(2):393–400.
23. Binder JR, Desai RH, Graves WW, Conant LL. Where is the semantic system? A critical review and meta-analysis of 120 functional neuroimaging studies. Cereb Cortex. 2009;19(12):2767–96.
24. Shin J, Rowley J, Chowdhury R, Jolicoeur P, Klein D, Grova C, Rosa-Neto P, Kobayashi E. Inferior longitudinal fasciculus' role in visual processing and language comprehension: a combined MEG-DTI study. Front Neurosci. 2019;13:875.
25. Mandonnet E, Nouet A, Gatignol P, Capelle L, Duffau H. Does the left inferior longitudinal fasciculus play a role in language? A brain stimulation study. Brain. 2007;130(3):623–9.
26. Ashtari M. Anatomy and functional role of the inferior longitudinal fasciculus: a search that has just begun. Develop Med Child Neurol. 2012;54(1):6–7.
27. Maffei C, Sarubbo S, Jovicich J. A missing connection: a review of the macrostructural anatomy and tractography of the acoustic radiation. Front Neuroanat. 2019;13:27.
28. Fenlon LR, Suarez R, Lynton Z, Richards LJ. The evolution, formation and connectivity of the anterior commissure. In Seminars in cell & developmental biology. Academic Press. 2021;118(1):50–9.
29. de Champfleur NM, Maldonado IL, Moritz-Gasser S, Machi P, Le Bars E, Bonafé A, Duffau H. Middle longitudinal fasciculus delineation within language pathways: a diffusion tensor imaging study in human. Eur J Radiol. 2013;82(1):151–7.
30. Bubb EJ, Metzler-Baddeley C, Aggleton JP. The cingulum bundle: anatomy, function, and dysfunction. Neurosci Biobehav Rev. 2018;1(92):104–27.
31. Louis D, Ohgaki H, Wiestler O, Cavenee WK. WHO classification of tumours of the central nervous system 4th edition revised volume. IARC. 2016;1:180–2.
32. Saur D, Kreher BW, Schnell S, Kümmerer D, Kellmeyer P, Vry MS, Umarova R, Musso M, Glauche V, Abel S, Huber W. Ventral and dorsal pathways for language. Proc Natl Acad Sci. 2008;105(46):18035–40.
33. Duffau H, Leroy M, Gatignol P. Cortico-subcortical organization of language networks in the right hemisphere: an electrostimulation study in left-handers. Neuropsychologia. 2008;46(14):3197–209.
34. Rodriguez A, Whitson J, Granger R. Derivation and analysis of basic computational operations of thalamocortical circuits. J Cogn Neurosci. 2004;16(5):856–77.
35. Phillips NS, Sanford RA, Helton KJ, Boop FA, Zou P, Tekautz T, Gajjar A, Ogg RJ. Diffusion tensor imaging of intraaxial tumors at the cervicomedullary and pontomedullary junctions: report of two cases. J Neurosurg Pediatr. 2005;103(6):557–62.
36. Epstein F, Wisoff JH. Surgical management of brain stem tumors of childhood and adolescence. Neurosurg Clin N Am. 1990;1(1):111–21.

Chapter 6
Intraoperative Adjuncts in Tumor Surgery

Rajesh Krishna Pathiyil

1. The disadvantages of frame-based stereotaxy when used intraoperatively include all of the following EXCEPT:

   (a) Interferes with the surgical field in major procedures.
   (b) Frame needs to be placed before imaging, and cannot be removed till the procedure is completed.
   (c) Accuracy is less compared to frameless neuronavigation machines.
   (d) It is difficult to change the trajectory intraoperatively.

   Answer: c

   Frame-based stereotaxy, which was earlier in use, has several limitations when used intraoperatively. The frame needs to be applied even before the acquisition of preoperative imaging which causes significant patient discomfort, especially in pediatric cases. The frame needs to remain in place throughout the entire duration of the procedure. This makes visualization and access to the surgical field difficult for the surgeon. There is no way to see the tip of the inserted needle in real-time. Planning needs to be done before the procedure and changing the trajectory intraoperatively is cumbersome.

   Frameless stereotaxy used in modern neuronavigation systems avoids the need for a rigid frame which creates problems both for the patient and the surgeon. The tip of the surgical instrument can be tracked in real-time, and the position can be projected on the preoperative imaging which is fed into the navigation system. The earlier systems which used ultrasonic waves, and later electromagnetic waves to locate the tip of instruments, were not accurate enough. Most of the current systems use optical digitalization technology using two infrared cameras, with improved accuracy.

R. K. Pathiyil (✉)
Department of Clinical Neurosciences, University of Calgary, Calgary, AB, Canada

Frameless neuronavigation systems have three essential components: (i) a preoperative image set of sufficient resolution that includes the area of interest and surface landmarks/ fiducials needed for registration, (ii) a trackable localizer tool, and (iii) a reference framework for the calculation of the relationship between the patient's anatomy and the preoperative image (like infrared cameras and reference array).

Framed stereotaxy remains the gold standard for stereotactic procedures, and has the best accuracy as the reference frame is fixed to the skull bone while taking preoperative imaging and no registration with additional hardware is involved, which is a step where inaccuracies can creep in. However, the present frameless neuronavigation systems have greatly improved accuracy, comparable to framed systems. The accuracy of surface registration can be improved by the use of fiducials. Scalp fiducials are easy to use and hence commonly employed, but this can lead to inaccuracies if the fiducials are placed over the mobile scalp or hair. Skull implanted fiducials help to get over this problem and have improved accuracy [1].

2. All of the following statements regarding errors in frameless stereotactic neuro-navigation systems are true EXCEPT:

   (a) In surface-based registration using the patient's facial features, the accuracy declines toward the occipital regions.
   (b) Ferromagnetic interference can lead to inaccuracies when electromagnetic device tracking technology is used.
   (c) Brain shifts do not always occur in the direction of gravity.
   (d) Once registration is completed using dynamic reference frames (DRFs), re-registration is always required for any change in the position of the patient's head.

   Answer: d

   In surface-based registration, the accuracy is best near the area where surface points are taken and declines as we move farther away from that area. While using the patient's facial features, the accuracy declines toward the occipital regions [2]. This can be reduced by supplementing surface-based registration with paired point registration using anatomical landmarks or scalp fiducials [1].

   Electromagnetic device tracking technology involves the generation of a magnetic field and the presence of coils in tracking devices. Hence, ferromagnetic interference can lead to inaccuracies when this technology is used [3, 4]. The advantages of this technology are that small coils can be attached to even suction devices and small catheters, and tracking does not require a free line of sight to be maintained.

   Neuronavigation systems assume a patient's head to be a rigid body. Once CSF is released after dural opening and the brain deflates, brain shift generally occurs vertically down towards the center of the earth. By positioning the head in such a way that the surgical trajectory is vertical, one needs to adjust for a shift only in one direction.

However, this explanation of brain shift is an oversimplification of the actual process. One should be aware that brain shift is a more complex spatiotemporal phenomenon that does not occur always in the direction of gravity. It is a slow phenomenon and continues to happen throughout the surgery. In addition to gravity and CSF loss, many other factors contribute to brain shifts including tissue manipulation, deformation of the tumor during resection, tumor size, and use of medications like mannitol [5]. The maximum brain shift occurs at the center of the craniotomy; the larger the craniotomy, the more the brain shift. The least deformation occurs towards the midline and skull base structures.

Other methods to reduce or compensate for brain shift include minimizing diuretics and hyperventilation, avoiding cyst puncture or ventricle puncture at the start of resection, attempting to remove the tumor en-bloc avoiding internal debulking, mechanically expanding the resection cavity with cottonoids if internal debulking is needed, resecting the most critical boundaries in the beginning when the shift is minimum, placing markers(fence posting) at critical boundaries before starting resection, and using intraoperative imaging modalities like ultrasound or MRI [1, 6].

Dynamic reference frames (DRFs) consist of a set of markers that are linked to the patient's head and usually attached to the patient's head holder. The registration remains valid as long as the head is moved along with the head holder without changing the position of the head relative to the DRF.

3. Which of the following statements regarding the incorporation of functional MRI (fMRI) and Diffusion Tensor Imaging (DTI) into standard navigation is TRUE?

   (a) Diffusion tractography helps to improve the extent of resection in high-grade gliomas, as compared to neuronavigation with standard sequences alone.
   (b) DTI conclusively distinguishes fiber tract disruption due to tumor infiltration from that due to vasogenic edema.
   (c) Precise language localization provided by fMRI obviates the need for awake surgery to localize these areas.
   (d) All of the above.

   Answer: a

   The addition of Diffusion Tensor Imaging (DTI) to standard neuronavigation has been shown to improve the extent of resection and improve survival in high-grade gliomas (level II evidence from a prospective RCT) [7]. DTI also helps to reduce postoperative deficits, resulting in better functional status. One of the limitations of DTI is that it cannot conclusively distinguish between fiber tract disruption due to tumor infiltration and vasogenic edema [8, 9].

Functional MRI (fMRI) has replaced the Wada test for language lateralization [10], but it has a sensitivity of less than 60% in precisely localizing the language areas [11–14]. fMRI shows activation of all the regions which are involved in the task being tested, but it does not tell us which region is functionally required, or which area is involved in what aspect of a particular function. On the other side, some areas which may be only transiently activated but functionally important, might not show up on fMRI. Awake surgery with intraoperative direct electrical stimulation (DES) remains the gold standard for language mapping.

4. Advantages of high field strength over low field strength intraoperative MRI (iMRI) include all of the following EXCEPT:

    (a) Better quality images.
    (b) Surgery need not be interrupted.
    (c) Allows multimodality imaging.
    (d) Can be used for routine diagnostic imaging while not in use.

    Answer: b

    Intraoperative MRI (iMRI) is in use in Neurosurgery since 1994. The most common use of iMRI is to assess the extent of tumor resection and to identify surrounding functioning neural tissues, avoiding damage to them. It also helps to compensate for brain shifts. iMRI can be used for targeted procedures like brain biopsy or cyst drainage.

    iMRI may be broadly divided into low field strength (0.5 T or less) and high field strength (1.5–3 T) devices. The first system developed by GE, which was nicknamed "the double doughnut", was designed in such a way that the surgeon operates between two vertically placed magnets, offering 0.5 T field strength. Though ergonomics of such an operative room setting were not optimum, it provided real-time imaging, unlike most high field strength systems that were marketed later. Low field strength iMRI devices are much less expensive than high field strength devices and may be operated with a local Faraday shielding, obviating the need to shield the walls of the operating room. While the lower resolution of low field strength iMRI might not be much of a problem in high-grade glioma surgeries, it might be troublesome in cases of low-grade gliomas where margins are not well-delineated [15].

    In addition to better image resolution, high-field systems also benefit from their ability to include other advanced techniques like MR spectroscopy, functional MRI, MR angiography, chemical shift imaging, and diffusion-weighted imaging [5]. But they come at a very high cost. Also, the installations are very heavy, putting a higher demand on the construction of the operating room. One advantage of high field strength iMRI is that it can be used for doing regular diagnostic MRI scans when not in use as an intraoperative adjunct.

    The main limitation of iMRI is its cost including the investment for MR compatible surgical instruments and modification of the operating room. It also results in interruption of surgery and longer operating times.

5. Which of the following statements regarding intraoperative ultrasound (iUS) is FALSE?

(a) Air between the probe and the brain results in artifacts.
(b) A large craniotomy is not always required for performing intraoperative ultrasound.
(c) iUS may delineate low-grade glioma margins better than MRI in some cases.
(d) iUS can't be integrated with a navigation system as they are registered on preoperative MRI or CT images.

Answer: d

The use of intraoperative ultrasound (iUS) was first described in Neurosurgery by Reid in 1978. iUS provides real-time updates regarding brain shifts and completeness of resection. It is less expensive compared to iMRI, but it involves a learning curve as Neurosurgeons are more used to interpreting MRI and CT images. Air bubbles and blood produce imaging artifacts, making it more difficult for the inexperienced. While using it, the air between the probe and the brain should be eliminated by filling up the cavity with saline and maintaining proper contact with the brain surface. Positioning the patient's head in such a way that the surgical trajectory is perpendicular to the floor, helps to keep the saline column from flowing out.

Though large craniotomies are preferred for iUS-guided resection of large tumors like diffuse insular gliomas, small burr hole probes are also available for doing procedures like iUS-guided brain biopsy.

Studies have shown that in non-enhancing gliomas, tumor margins may be delineated better by iUS than from the T2/FLAIR hyperintensities of the preoperative MRI. Many non-enhancing gliomas which are categorised as moderately delineated on preoperative MRI have relatively well-delineated margins on iUS images [16, 17].

Sweeps of 2D ultrasound scans with probes attached to a trackable localizer can be reconstructed into 3D volumes and then superimposed onto the preoperative MRI images in the Neuronavigation system. This helps the surgeon to appreciate the orientation of the images acquired by 3D ultrasound better. It also helps us to estimate the brain shift that has occurred after initial registration [18]. The navigation accuracy of 3D ultrasound-based neuronavigation is comparable to standard MR image-based neuronavigation systems [19]. Navigated iUS have been shown to improve the extent of resection in gliomas while reducing morbidity [16, 20, 21].

6. Which of the following statements is TRUE regarding contrast-enhanced ultrasonography (CEUS)?

(a) The contrast agent consists of thin-shelled microbubbles.
(b) It is contraindicated in patients with renal impairment.
(c) It has not shown to be of much use in intraoperative neuro sonography.
(d) Low-grade gliomas appear hypoechoic on post-contrast ultrasound scan images.

Answer: a

Intraoperative contrast-enhanced ultrasonography (CEUS) is useful in high-lighting the tumor better when compared with standard B-mode imaging and showing its perfusion patterns. The afferent and efferent blood vessels can be identified. CEUS also helps to define tumor margins better, especially in high-grade gliomas and also helps to differentiate viable and necrotic areas of the tumor. The contrast agent is made up of microbubbles of air or inert gas encapsulated in a layer of proteins or polymers, which are typically 5 μm in diameter and can therefore be transported into the smallest capillaries and across the lungs. The passage across the lungs allows imaging of the arterial system with a venous injection [22]. It doesn't have major adverse effects. The contrast agent remains purely intravascular and does not extravasate. Elimination of microbubbles occurs through fragmentation and diffusion and is not dependent on renal or hepatic mechanisms [23]. In general, glioblastomas, metastases, and meningiomas appear hyperechoic on CEUS. Low-grade gliomas and anaplastic astrocytomas appear isoechoic to mildly hyperechoic [22].

7. Which of the following statements regarding ultrasound probes is TRUE?

   (a) High-frequency probes have higher depth penetration.
   (b) All the probes used in intraoperative ultrasonography have fixed frequencies.
   (c) A linear array probe covers a wider area at a distance away from the probe compared to a phased array probe.
   (d) Spatial resolution normal to the scan plane (elevation resolution) is a key parameter in 3D reconstruction.

   Answer: d

   The iUS image quality depends on its spatial resolution, which in turn depends on the frequency of the probe used. High-frequency probes have higher resolution and better image quality but do not have good depth penetration. Lower frequency probes have better depth penetration but show poorer image resolution. Hence higher frequency probes are better suited for surface imaging while low-frequency ones are for depth imaging.

   One of the reasons why iUS image quality has improved over the recent years is because the probes can be electronically tuned for a range of frequencies, which provides optimum image quality at multiple depths. The probe commonly used in brain surgeries is a 5 MHz probe which can usually be electronically tuned over a range of frequencies from 4 MHz to 8 MHz. This gives optimum images at a depth of 2.5–6 cm where most supratentorial lesions are seen. For surface cerebral lesions or lesions in the posterior fossa, medulla or spinal cord a high frequency 10 MHz probe can be used which provides the best image quality at 0.5–4 cm depths.

   Linear transducers have piezoelectric crystals arranged linearly and the shape of the beam is rectangular. The extension of the image is limited to the width of the probe. Its near-field resolution is good and is optimal for imaging superficial lesions where the bone is removed over the lesion. Hockey stick probes used in Neurosurgery are modifications of linear probes with a smaller footprint.

In a convex transducer, the piezoelectric crystal arrangement is curvilinear. The beam shape is convex and the transducer is good for in-depth examinations. Smaller micro-convex craniotomy probes with smaller footprints of about 3 cm, and operating over a wide range of frequencies of 5–13 MHz are available in the market, and this provides optimum image quality for most neurosurgical procedures, including the acquisition of 3D ultrasound images.

Phased array probes have a small footprint and low frequencies. It consists of arrays of ultrasound transducers that are fired multiple times with different degrees of steering to create an image. The beam point is narrow but it fans out depending on the applied frequency. The beam shape is almost triangular and the near-field resolution is poor.

As mentioned earlier, spatial resolution determines the image quality. The resolution along the transmitted beam, which is called the radial resolution, equals approximately the transmitted pulse length. The resolution normal to the beam is called lateral resolution. It is equal to the beamwidth. Elevation resolution is the one that is normal to the scan plane. The elevation resolution is a key parameter for the 3D reconstruction which is done by putting many 2D frames together [18].

8. The advantages of intraoperative 3D ultrasound compared to iMRI include all of the following EXCEPT:

(a) 3D ultrasound is less expensive.
(b) It gives better orientation compared to iMRI.
(c) It is faster to acquire.
(d) Surgery is interrupted to a lesser extent.

Answer: b

Even the best ultrasound machine is much cheaper than setting up an iMRI facility of the lowest field strength. It does not require additional special installations or special compatible instruments. The time for acquisition of a 3D iUS interval scan during surgery is around 2–4 min, and is real-time, without much interruption to the surgery. Newer high-end ultrasound devices have been reported to be comparable to or even better than MRI in delineating tumor margins, especially with non-enhancing gliomas [16, 17].

But there is a learning curve for interpreting iUS images, as Neurosurgeons are more familiar with CT and MRI images. The images are obtained in unfamiliar planes and not in the conventional axial, sagittal, and coronal planes. The non-availability of the wholesome view of the brain also makes interpretation of iUS images difficult. Superimposing 3D iUS images onto the preoperative MRI images in the neuronavigation system helps to improve our orientation while interpreting these images. Some authors also feel that iUS increases the chances of infection as compared to iMRI as the former is not a contactless technique.

9. Which of the following statements regarding intraoperative sonoelastography is TRUE?

   (a) Shear-wave elastography (SWE) is a qualitative evaluation, whereas axial strain elastography (SE) provides more quantitative data.
   (b) All cerebral metastases are stiffer than normal brain parenchyma.
   (c) Color coding in sonoelastography is usually done in such a way that greenish shades indicate softer tissues while stiffer areas are shown in red.
   (d) Margins of low-grade gliomas are more discernable in B-mode ultrasound scans than by using sonoelastography.

Answer: c

Sonoelastography is a tactile imaging technique that transcribes manual palpation into ultrasonography images. It represents the mechanical property of the tissue, defined by the relationship between stress (applied force) and strain (proportional deformation), which is extremely variable between different tissues. This allows for excellent contrast.

Two frequently used techniques in Neurosurgery are shear wave elastography (SWE) and axial-strain elastography (SE). SWE uses focused ultrasound to induce very small tissue displacements; this generates shear waves that propagate in the orthogonal plane to tissue displacement. SWE is a quantitative technique that measures the absolute stiffness of tissues, but it is not available in many commercially available systems. On the other hand, SE is a commonly available qualitative sonoelastography method that involves the acquisition of ultrasound scans before and after applying a deformation force. Deformation can be obtained either with multiple cycles of gentle pressure release on the US probe or by utilizing tissue motion caused by brain arterial pulsations [24]. It measures relative (not absolute) tissue stiffness. In SE, the information is obtained real-time, whereas quantitative SWE data requires post-processing; hence SE might be easier to use in an operating room, whereas SWE provides more accurate information for research purposes.

Low-grade gliomas tend to be stiffer than normal brain parenchyma, while most high-grade gliomas are softer. In most cases, the glioma margins are better delineated using sonoelastography than in B-mode scans, both in low-grade and high-grade gliomas.

Some metastases are stiffer than the brain (renal cell carcinoma, colon carcinoma), while some others are softer than the brain (endometrial cancer, lung cancer). Hemangioblastomas can be softer than the brain, while germ cell tumors and lymphomas are stiffer.

Sonoelastography has been reported to show epileptogenic lesions like focal cortical dysplasias which are not even seen in MRI [25].

10. Which of the following intraoperative modalities helps to compensate for brain shifts by assessing cortical surface deformation?

    (a) Intraoperative 3D ultrasound.
    (b) Laser Range Scanner.
    (c) StereoVision.
    (d) b and c.

   Answer: d

   Modalities like Laser Range Scanners (LRS) and StereoVision acquire the intraoperative cortical surface deformation which is then integrated into a pre-computed patient-specific biomedical model to estimate the volumetric deformation. Stereovision is the process of extracting 3D information from digital images taken by two cameras displaced horizontally from one another to obtain two different views of the same scene. The reconstructed images are displayed over the patient's preoperative images in the physical space. Stereovision systems can be coupled to operating microscopes. This helps to estimate intraoperative brain shifts in real-time without interrupting the surgery. This technology is relatively less expensive and contactless [5, 26].

11. Which of the following is a telesurgical robot used in Neurosurgery?

    (a) ROSA.
    (b) NeuroMate.
    (c) NeuroArm.
    (d) SpineAssist.

   Answer: c

   The surgical robots were first used in the field of Neurosurgery. PUMA- 200 robot which was originally designed for industrial use, was used for CT-guided needle biopsy. The first FDA-approved robot was NeuroMate. The robots currently in use are classified into three categories [27]:

   (i) **Telesurgical robot (Master-slave)**—In this type, the surgeon controls the robot from a remote workstation outside the operating room. It can even provide tactile feedback to the surgeon. e.g.: NeuroArm

   (ii) **Supervisory surgeon-controlled robot**—In this type, the robot assists the surgeon and helps to improve precision. The main use of these robots has been taking stereotactic biopsies in brain tumors and improving the precision of screw placement in the spine. e.g.: PUMA- 200, Minerva, Pathfinder, SpineAssist.

   (iii) **Handheld shared/controlled systems**—In these systems, the surgeon and the robot jointly control the instruments. The precision contributed by the robotic system and the manual dexterity and manipulative skills contributed by the Neurosurgeon leads to better instrument handling. The robot can also mark out the safe zone, which prevents the surgeon from straying and injuring important structures. It can also reduce surgeon's hand tremors and fatigue. eg: Steady hand system, Evolution 1, ROSA.

12. Disadvantages of using robots in Neurosurgery include all of the following EXCEPT:

    (a) Reduced range of manipulation.
    (b) Impairs situational awareness.
    (c) Surgeon's hands tend to get fatigued earlier with hand-held systems.
    (d) Steep learning curve.

    Answer: c

    Hand held surgical robots reduce hand fatigue and surgeon's tremors. They also serve as a resting stand which avoids unnecessary straying, thus preventing accidental injury to critical structures.

    The main difficulties in using robotic systems are that they are expensive and have a steeper learning curve. Most of the systems do not provide tactile feedback to the surgeon. It can reduce the surgeon's situational awareness, and this can lead to errors during the procedure. The robotic arms may also have a limited range of movements and dexterity [27].

13. Which intraoperative modality is the gold standard while operating upon tumors near eloquent brain regions?

    (a) Intraoperative fluorescence with 5-ALA.
    (b) Neuronavigation with fMRI and DTI data integrated.
    (c) Awake surgery with cortical and subcortical mapping.
    (d) Robot-assisted tumor resection.

    Answer: c

    Awake surgery with cortical and subcortical mapping using direct electrical stimulation (DES) remains the gold-standard technique to improve the extent of resection and reduce morbidity while resecting tumors near eloquent brain areas. Monitoring brain functions other than motor function, like language and complex neurocognitive functions, requires the patient to be awake. Awake brain mapping has led to an expansion of surgical targets to those areas which were previously considered to be surgically inaccessible. It has also led to the appreciation of the phenomenon of cortical plasticity and has led to the rejection of some of the classical localization theories of brain organization.

14. All of the following statements are true regarding awake intraoperative mapping EXCEPT:

    (a) Modalities like language and higher neuropsychological functions can only be tested during awake mapping.
    (b) General anesthesia with muscle relaxants should be administered in the event of intraoperative seizures.
    (c) Awake surgery with intraoperative mapping allows supratotal resection of tumors.
    (d) Awake mapping allows testing of the volitional aspects of movement.

    Answer: b

Except for the primary motor cortex and motor tracts, mapping of any functional brain area requires the patient to be awake. Even for the primary motor cortex, spatial fidelity for mapping is better when awake. Awake mapping allows for testing of volitional aspects of movement, for instance, negative motor areas in supplementary motor and parietal regions [14, 28, 29]. Subcortical stimulation of areas underlying SMA can induce deficits of complex motor coordination like bimanual coordination or coordination of contralateral upper and lower limbs, which will be missed if the mapping is not done in an awake state.

Glioma should be looked upon as a disease of the brain, rather than a discrete tumor entity. The fact that gliomas extend well beyond the radiological margins is well appreciated, especially in low-grade tumors. So, the current concept is to map the functional boundaries with DES and resect the tumor beyond its 'radiological margins' until 'functional margins' are reached (supratotal resection). This improves the extent of resection while reducing morbidity, thus improving the progression-free survival as well as the quality of life of these patients. Awake mapping should become the rule rather than an exception.

Seizures occurring during awake mapping are generally aborted by cessation of stimulus and irrigating the cortical surface with ice-cold saline. The occurrence of seizures can be reduced by starting with a lower current strength, and avoiding continuous or repeated stimulation over the same gyrus (which leads to temporal summation). Using muscle electrodes to monitor motor response instead of looking for overt muscle contraction, obviates the need for higher current strengths.

15. Which of the following patients is NOT a good candidate for awake mapping?

    (a) Pediatric patients.
    (b) Patients with contralateral limb power less than 3/5.
    (c) >25% error rate on preoperative language tests.
    (d) All of the above.

    Answer: d

    Patients with already existing major deficits might not yield reliable information on mapping with DES. Patients with less than antigravity strength in the muscles to be monitored or those with significant preoperative language deficit (error rate > 25% in preoperative language tests) are not good candidates for mapping. Pediatric patients, as well as patients who do not co-operate well for awake mapping like those with major neurocognitive impairment or anxiety, should not be offered awake craniotomy [14]. Using awake mapping in this scenario can be counterproductive. Proper patient selection is key to successful awake surgery. Patient's co-operation is imperative. If the patient becomes uncooperative or restless, there should be an alternative option to anesthetize him before proceeding; otherwise, the surgeon might unnecessarily hurry through the procedure resulting in a suboptimal resection or additional morbidity. Asleep monitoring or a more conservative resection using anatomical landmarks should be considered for these patients.

In prolonged surgeries, as in diffuse insular gliomas, patients might get tired and monitoring higher neurocognitive functions might become unreliable as the surgery proceeds. In these cases, a 'asleep-awake-asleep' approach is a good option where the patient is asleep till craniotomy is performed, made awake while doing dural opening, and then made to sleep again after necessary functions are mapped. This improves patient cooperation. One should consider dissecting tumor margins close to areas that require a high level of patient cooperation and alertness while monitoring at the earlier stages of surgery [30]. In cases of tumors where torrential bleeding is expected intraoperatively, anesthetic management might be difficult with the patient remaining awake.

16. Which of the following statements regarding language mapping is TRUE?

    (a) Language mapping usually starts with a demonstration of speech arrest over the ventral premotor cortex.
    (b) While doing picture naming, it is important to record responses in complete sentences.
    (c) In multilingual patients, cotical representations of the same function for different languages can be distinct.
    (d) All of the above.

    Answer: d

    Language mapping usually starts with simple number counting and demonstrating speech arrest over the ventral premotor cortex. This lies within the anterior precentral gyrus, and not over the classically described Broca's area which is in the pars opercularis and pars triangularis of the inferior frontal gyrus [14, 31]. This also helps to identify the stimulation threshold for that particular patient while doing further language mapping.

    The next test performed is picture naming. DES over the cortex is given just before changing the picture. Each stimulation-associated picture can be alternated with one presented without stimulation, which acts as an internal control. One should look for speech arrest, anomia, phonemic or semantic paraphasia, or perseveration. One should insist that the patient responds in complete sentences, to differentiate anomia from speech arrest.

    Bilinguals have language-specific sites as well as shared language sites. Studies showed that posterior regions possess language-specific sites for secondary language, whereas anterior regions generally lack such sites. It was also shown that secondary language areas in bilinguals are restricted from certain perisylvian areas [32]. Hence it is necessary to map both the languages in bilinguals.

17. Which of the following responses is seen on stimulation of inferior fronto-occipital fasciculus (IFOF) in the dominant hemisphere?

    (a) Semantic paraphasia.
    (b) Phonological paraphasia.

(c) Speech arrest.

(d) Reading difficulty.

Answer: a

The subcortical language pathways consist of dorsal and ventral pathways. The dorsal stream, which is the phonological pathway, consists of the arcuate fasciculus and superior longitudinal fasciculus (SLF III). The ventral semantic stream is formed by inferior fronto-occipital fasciculus (IFOF). IFOF, which is the longest fiber bundle in humans, has a broader role in multimodal semantic processing. On stimulation, the superficial layer of IFOF produces semantic paraphasia while performing picture naming, whereas the deeper layer causes disorders in semantic association tasks.

Inferior longitudinal fasciculus (ILF) connects anterior temporal and occipital lobes. The posterior part of ILF has a critical role in reading. Intraoperative stimulation of posterior ILF elicits reproducible visual paraphasia and dyslexia [14].

In addition to white matter tracts, mapping of deep nuclei can also be done while testing for language functions. Stimulation of the caudate nucleus elicits perseveration while doing picture naming task. Stimulation of the lentiform nucleus produces dysarthria.

18. All of the following statements are true regarding subcortical monitoring during insular glioma resection EXCEPT:

(a) Eliciting phonological paraphasia marks the deeper limit of resection in the temporal stem.

(b) Posterior deeper limit of resection is the posterior limb of the internal capsule.

(c) Resection of tumor involving uncinate fasciculus, anterior ILF, and anterior MLF will not produce significant postoperative dysfunction.

(d) Lentiform nucleus, stimulation of which produces articulatory disturbances, marks the medial limit of resection.

Answer: a

The deeper limits of resection in insular glioma are [30, 33]:

(i) Posterior limb of the internal capsule (pyramidal tract) in the posterior insular quadrant.

(ii) The dorsal language pathway, which involves arcuate fasciculus/superior longitudinal fasciculus complex in the depths of the frontal lobe; stimulation elicits speech apraxia, phonological paraphasia, and repetition difficulty

(iii) The ventral semantic pathway (IFOF) in the anterior part of the insula marks the limit of resection in the temporal stem. Stimulation of IFOF in the dominant hemisphere elicits semantic paraphasia. In the non-dominant hemisphere, it elicits non-verbal semantic disturbances. Ventral IFOF compensates for the functions of uncinate fasciculus, anterior ILF, and anterior MLF. Hence tumors involving these tracts can be resected safely without much post-operative deficit.

(iv) The lentiform nucleus forms the deeper limit behind the temporal stem. It can be identified during surgery by its characteristic nutmeg appearance. It has a role in articulation planning and stimulation of this area induces articulatory disturbances.

(v) The anterior perforated substance with the lenticulostriate vessels, medially.

19. In which of the following scenarios is somatosensory evoked potential (SSEP) least useful?

(a) To monitor during resection of intramedullary tumors.
(b) To monitor cervical cord compression or brachial plexus stretch during positioning of the patient for surgery.
(c) To identify motor cortex during cranial surgeries.
(d) To monitor during resection of posteriorly placed intradural extramedullary tumors.

Answer: a

For SSEP monitoring, peripheral sensory nerves are stimulated and the response is measured along the sensory pathway or the primary somatosensory cortex. The recorded activity primarily reflects the conduction along the posterior column sensation pathways. The major cortical responses recorded correspond to the thalamocortical projections to the primary sensory cortex. So SSEP helps to monitor the sensory pathway along the peripheral nerves, spinal cord, brain stem, and subcortical structures.

SSEP is useful in monitoring during spinal cord surgeries. Generally, a decrease in amplitude by 50% or an increase in peak latency by 10% is considered to be significant. Unlike motor evoked potential (MEP) monitoring which cannot be monitored continuously, SSEP can be monitored continuously throughout the surgery without interruption. One of the disadvantages of SSEP in spinal cord surgeries is that motor deficits are known to occur even with preserved SSEP responses. This is because SSEP monitors the posterior spinal cord supplied by the posterior spinal artery, whereas motor tracts are located anteriorly in the area supplied by the anterior spinal artery. SSEP (with peripheral sensory nerve stimulation) is also not sensitive to detecting individual root injury, as multiple roots contribute to the cortical response; CMAPs recorded during MEP are more sensitive to detecting root injury. Dermatomal evoked potential (DEP), obtained by stimulating each dermatome, is a more specific response for each root, but it is not commonly used.

SSEP also helps to identify physiological insults like hypotension, nerve compression, nerve stretch, or cervical spinal cord compression that might occur during patient positioning.

SSEP can be used to identify the motor cortex by phase reversal of the response (response changes from positive to negative) which can be demonstrated by placing cortical strip electrodes across the central sulcus [34].

20. Which of the following statements regarding H reflex is FALSE?

(a) It monitors sensory and motor components of the nerve, as well as the spinal grey matter.
(b) It is the electrical equivalent of deep tendon reflex.
(c) It is less sensitive than SSEP to detect spinal cord injury cephalad to the level of the monitored nerve.
(d) None of the above.

Answer: c

When a peripheral motor nerve is stimulated, the initial compound muscle action potential (CMAP) recorded from the muscle is called M-response. The stimulation of sensory fibers in the nerve causes impulses to travel proximally, which passes through the spinal reflex arc and travels back along the motor fibers, creating a response called H-reflex. The stimulation also produces a depolarization that travels along the motor nerve centrally towards the cord and is then reflected, producing a response, which is called an F wave.

The suprasegmental tracts influence the spinal reflex response and hence alter the H-reflex. These changes have been shown to appear earlier than SSEP changes [34].

21. All of the following complications have been reported with MEP monitoring except:

(a) Sore muscles.
(b) Neuropsychiatric disease.
(c) Kindling.
(d) Cardiac arrhythmias.

Answer: b

Sore muscles and tongue lacerations are the most common complications of transcranial MEP monitoring. There are also reports of cardiac arrhythmias, scalp burns, and jaw fractures. Kindling is direct cortical thermal injury, which is an extremely rare complication [34].

22. The advantages of D-wave monitoring include all of the following EXCEPT:

(a) Altered little by anesthetics.
(b) Differentiate laterality of injury.
(c) Not affected by muscle relaxants.
(d) More sensitive than SSEP to motor tract injury.

Answer: b

Transcranial stimulation of motor tracts produces a wave of depolarization that can be recorded using electrodes placed in the spinal epidural or subdural space. This is called D wave (direct wave). I waves (indirect waves) are a series of smaller waves that follows the D wave. I waves are a result of additional trans-synaptic activation of internuncial neurons in the cortex. D and I waves summate over the anterior horn cells, producing a peripheral response (CMAP).

As the D wave is measured before the first synapse, it is the least affected by anesthetic agents. Obviously, muscle relaxants do not alter this response. But the epidural/subdural electrodes can record potentials from either side, hence not very useful in differentiating the laterality of the injury.

In contrast to SSEP monitoring which monitors the posterior column supplied by the posterior spinal arteries, D waves represent the motor tracts located in the anterior spinal artery territory and hence are more valuable in predicting postoperative motor deficits [34].

23. Which of the following brainstem auditory evoked response (BAER) waves can be lost even in patients with preserved hearing?

    (a) Wave I.
    (b) Wave III.
    (c) Wave V.
    (d) None of the above.

    Answer: c

    Brainstem auditory evoked response (BAER) refers to the auditory responses recorded from cranial nerve VIII and the brain stem usually during the first 10 ms after auditory stimulation. It has five peaks labeled from I to V, of which I, III, and V are more prominent.

    I—extracranial cranial nerve VIII.
    II—cochlear nucleus.
    III—superior olivary complex (lower pons).
    IV—lateral lemniscus.
    V—inferior colliculus (midbrain).

    BAER is used for monitoring auditory nerve and brain stem injury during posterior fossa tumor surgeries. Loss of peaks or prolongation of interpeak latencies points towards damage at corresponding locations. Changes in wave V have the least correlation with the outcome as it can be lost due to desynchronization in the pathways even when hearing is preserved.

    Response to auditory stimulation recorded over the sensory cortex is termed mid latency auditory evoked response. It is usually used as an index of anesthetic effect [34].

24. What is the normal latency for facial nerve EMG response when the nerve is stimulated in the CP angle?

    (a) 3–4 ms.
    (b) 6–8 ms.
    (c) 14–16 ms.
    (d) 30–32 ms.

    Answer: b

Electromyography (EMG) is commonly used in neurosurgery for intraoperative monitoring. Here muscle responses are utilized to monitor neural tracts. Electrical responses can be played through a loudspeaker which provides real-time feedback to the operating surgeon.

Nerve irritation can produce responses, which can be short bursts or long trains. Short bursts ("blurps"), which last less than 200 ms, represent synchronous motor discharges when multiple axons of the nerve are stimulated simultaneously by retraction, mechanical or thermal irritation. Long trains of continuous discharges ("popcorn" or "bomber" sounds) lasting 1 to 30 s or more, represent impending nerve injury due to compression, traction, or ischemia.

Intentional stimulation with low intensity (0.5–5 mA), short duration (0.5–1 ms) current is used to check the continuity of the nerve or to locate the nerve fascicles as in cerebellopontine angle tumor surgeries.

Unlike cortical responses, EMG responses -spontaneous as well as in reponse to nerve stimulation—are resistant to the effects of anesthetics but are affected by neuromuscular blockade [34].

When stimulated in the CP angle, the normal latency for facial nerve response is about 6–8 ms while that of trigeminal nerve responses is 3–4 ms. This helps in differentiating true signals from the facial muscles from the artifacts produced from strong contractions of temporalis or masseter.

25. Which of the following statements regarding navigated transcranial magnetic stimulation (nTMS) for cortical mapping is TRUE?

    (a) It is noninvasive.
    (b) nTMS hot spots can be utilized to improve the accuracy of DTI.
    (c) Motor maps generated using nTMS were found to be more concordant with DES than the language maps.
    (d) All of the above.

    Answer: d

    Transcranial magnetic stimulation (TMS) is a non-invasive method that involves using a single pulsed magnetic field to activate small volumes of the brain close to the cortical surface. TMS software can be integrated with the navigation device (nTMS), which allows precise delivery of magnetic fields for cortical stimulation. nTMS motor maps have been demonstrated to correlate well with DES [35, 36]. Language maps generated using nTMS also correlate with maps generated by DES, but they are not as concordant as in the case of motor maps. Negative language mapping is more important as it was found to correlate well in both modalities. In contrast to single pulses of the magnetic field used in TMS motor mapping, language mapping utilizes short bursts of TMS pulses called repetitive TMS.

    nTMS generated primary motor cortex hot spots have been utilized to generate highly accurate tractography of corticospinal tracts. Similar utility was also demonstrated with regards to language subcortical tracts. nTMS was also shown to be useful in mapping the primary visual cortex. It is also being tried for mapping complex neuropsychological functions involving frontal and parietal lobes [37]. Maps generated using nTMS can be generated preoperatively. This helps to plan the surgical approach well in advance.

TMS-induced seizure is seen in <1% of cases. US FDA recommends that TMS should not be used for preoperative mapping in patients with poorly controlled seizures (>1 seizure/week). Other complications reported include pain, headache, and high-frequency hearing loss [37].

26. Which of the following responses is least affected by inhalational anesthetic agents?

    (a) Muscle CMAPs.
    (b) D wave.
    (c) Cortical SSEP.
    (d) BAER.

    Answer: b

    Anesthetic agents act to reduce synaptic transmission. In SSEP, the first synapses occur at the level of nucleus cuneatus and gracilis. So, the anesthetic drugs have little effect on SSEPs recorded at the level of the cervical spine. Similarly, during MEP monitoring, D-waves are not affected by anesthetic agents as there are no synapses involved, whereas the I wave and muscle CMAPs are reduced. In general, inhalational anesthetic agents have the most profound influence on slowing synaptic transmission, hence total intravenous anesthesia (TIVA) is preferred, especially when MEPs are monitored. Propofol is currently the most common sedative used in TIVA, although depression of MEPs can occur at higher doses. Ketamine has an enhancement effect on cortical SSEP responses and CMAPs in MEP monitoring. Hence, the use of ketamine along with propofol helps to reduce the depressant effect of the latter. Opioids cause only mild depression of responses. Dexmedetomidine also appears to have minimal effect on the responses. Thiopental and midazolam cause long-lasting depression in MEP responses. Etomidate can cause high cortical excitability, resulting in increased amplitude of cortical sensory responses, hence has been used with SSEP monitoring and not commonly with MEP monitoring. Neuromuscular blockade interferes with MEP and EMG monitoring. A technique called post-tetanic MEPs may be useful in patients in whom partial paralysis is desired. In this technique, a tetanic stimulus is delivered to the peripheral nerve before the MEPs to enhance the responses. Other factors including hypoxemia, hypotension, hypothermia, hypoglycemia, electrolyte abnormalities, anemia, and raised intracranial tension, also affect the responses during monitoring.

27. What is the dose and route of 5-aminolevulinic acid administered for intraoperative tumor fluorescence?

   (a) 20 mg /kg orally.
   (b) 20 mg/kg slow iv.
   (c) 2 mg/kg orally.
   (d) 2 mg/kg iv.

   Answer: a

   5-aminolevulinic acid (5-ALA) is a precursor in hemoglobin synthesis. It is metabolized inside tumor cells into fluorescent protoporphyrin IX (PpIX) which emits a red-violet fluorescence under blue light. Solid red fluorescence corresponds to highly proliferating tumor tissue, whereas vague pink fluorescence corresponds to the infiltrating tumor cells in the transitional area between the tumor and normal brain. Necrotic areas in high-grade gliomas do not fluoresce. It differs from other fluorescing agents like fluorescein, which penetrates malignant glioma via the defective blood-brain barrier. 5- ALA is administered orally at a dose of 20 mg/kg dissolved in 50 ml of water about 3 h (range 2–4 h) before induction of anesthesia.

   Stummer et al. reported that the rates of complete resection as well as 6-month progression-free survival in malignant glioma were doubled with the use of 5-ALA [38]. Another advantage of intraoperative tumor fluorescence when compared to other modalities like iMRI and intraoperative ultrasound is that it does not interrupt the surgery.

   Disadvantages of 5-ALA [39]:

   (i) Expensive
   (ii) Skin reactions (photosensitivity). Exposure to sunlight or strong room light should be avoided for 24 h after administration of 5-ALA.
   (iii) Difficult to operate continuously under blue light.
   (iv) Many other pathologies also show fluorescence.

28. Which of the following fluoresce least after 5-ALA administration?

   (a) Low-grade glioma.
   (b) Grade I meningioma.
   (c) Cerebral inflammation.
   (d) Cerebral metastasis.

   Answer: a

   The utility of 5-ALA tumor fluorescence is well studied for high-grade gliomas (level I evidence) where it has a sensitivity of around 85%. It is not useful in low-grade glioma resection where the sensitivity was reported from 0 to 16% in various studies. 5-ALA is a good marker of tumor anaplasticity. Meningiomas also show fluorescence. Though grade II/III meningiomas have increased sensitivity to 5-ALA tumor fluorescence, approximately 70% of grade I meningiomas also fluoresce. The sensitivity of ALA fluorescence for cerebral metastasis is lower (54%). Studies have also shown that PpIX accumulates in peritumor tissues around the metastases emitting a vague fluorescence with high false-positive rates [40]. Fluorescence is also seen in areas of cerebral inflammation, fungal and bacterial abscesses, CNS lymphoma, radiation necrosis, multiple sclerosis, and some normal brain tissues like ventricular ependyma [41].

29. Which of the following statements regarding 5-ALA tumor fluorescence is FALSE?

    (a) Prolonged exposure to the microscope light can result in photobleaching of porphyrins resulting in reduced fluorescence.
    (b) 5-ALA obviates the need for electrophysiological mapping and monitoring.
    (c) If surgery is delayed, but not beyond 12 h of 5-ALA administration, repeat administration of the dye is not required.
    (d) Neon ambient lighting can interfere with fluorescence signal.

    Answer: b

    It was shown that 5-ALA tumor fluorescence decayed to 36% in 25 minutes for violet-blue, and 87 minutes for white light [42]. This happens only in exposed areas of the tumor. Fluorescence may be refreshed by suction and removal of superficial cell layers.

    5-ALA fluorescence is more sensitive than MRI in delineating tumor margins. Fluorescing tumor volume is usually larger than the volume in contrast-enhanced MRI sequences. The tumor infiltrating into functioning brain areas also fluoresce. Studies have shown that even though 5-ALA improves the extent of resection, there can be a higher incidence of neurological deficits when this modality is used alone for gliomas near eloquent areas. Awake intraoperative monitoring is required while operating near functional brain areas to reduce deficits [40].

    The peak plasma levels of PpIX are reached 7–8 h after oral administration [43]; excellent tumor fluorescence is obtained for at least 9 h. Then it rapidly declines over the next 20 h and is not detectable by 48 h. If the surgery is delayed by more than 12 h, surgery should be preferably re-scheduled for the next day or later. There is no robust data available on the safety of repeat administration of ALA on the same day.

    Neon ambient lighting contains substantial red and infrared light. Red wavelengths are selectively amplified by the detection equipment. This leads to reddish discoloration of non-tumor tissue, which is otherwise normally perceived as being blue. Standard surgical lights are usually filtered in the red and infrared wavelengths. The operating rooms have to be darkened for daylight.

30. All of the following statements regarding sodium fluorescein tumor fluorescence are true EXCEPT:

    (a) Tumor fluorescence can be seen under white light.
    (b) Tumor fluorescence is best visualized under blue light.
    (c) Sodium fluorescein helps to identify dural tail in meningiomas.

(d) For tumor fluorescence sodium fluorescein needs to be administered intrathecally once the patient is inside the operating room.

Answer: d

Fluorescein is a red or dark orange colored powder which turns yellow when mixed with water. Sodium fluorescein is relatively inexpensive and easily accessible, and helps to improve the percentage of complete resection similar to 5-ALA [44]. Once injected into the blood it leaks into the tissues where blood-brain barrier is lacking. It is administered at a dose of 2–20 mg/kg intravenously [39]. Though the dye is best viewed using a yellow light filter (Y560) which allows blue light to pass through, higher doses have been shown to exhibit good tumor fluorescence in white light as well [39, 45]. In addition to high-grade gliomas, its use has also been reported with other brain tumors like cerebral metastases, PCNSL, meningiomas, craniopharyngiomas, acoustic neuromas, and pituitary adenomas. It has been shown to be helpful in identifying the dural tail of meningiomas which could represent tumor infiltration [39, 46].

Fluorescein sodium can cause transient yellowish discoloration of skin and urine. It has been reported to cause intraoperative hypotension and rarely, anaphylactic reaction [47, 48]. It should be used with caution in patients having hepatic or renal dysfunction, pulmonary spasm, and a history of allergic reactions to contrast dyes.

Intrathecal administration of fluorescein is commonly used in cases of CSF leak to identify the site of the leak intraoperatively.

Test your learning and check your understanding of this book's contents: use the "Springer Nature Flashcards" app to access questions using https://sn.pub/3HwHCw To use the app, please follow the instructions in Chap. 1.

References

1. Missios S, Barnett GH. Surgical navigation of brain tumours. In: Youmans and Winn Neurological Surgery. 7th ed. 2017. p. 973–80.
2. Raabe A, Krishnan R, Wolff R, Hermann E, Zimmermann M, Seifert V, et al. Laser surface scanning for patient registration in intracranial image-guided surgery. Neurosurgery [Internet]. 2002;50(4):797–803.
3. Birkfellner W, Watzinger F, Wanschitz F, Enislidis G, Kollmann C, Rafolt D, et al. Systematic distortions in magnetic position digitizers. Med Phys [Internet]. 1998;25(11):2242–8. https://onlinelibrary.wiley.com/doi/full/10.1118/1.598425
4. Hummel J, Figl M, Birkfellner W, Bax MR, Shahidi R, Maurer CR, et al. Evaluation of a new electromagnetic tracking system using a standardized assessment protocol. Phys Med Biol [Internet]. 2006;51(10):N205. https://iopscience.iop.org/article/10.1088/0031-9155/51/10/N01
5. Bayer S, Maier A, Ostermeier M, Fahrig R. Intraoperative imaging modalities and compensation for brain shift in tumor resection surgery. Int J Biomed Imaging [Internet] 2017. /pmc/articles/PMC5476838/

6. Yoshikawa K, Kajiwara K, Morioka J, Fujii M, Tanaka N, Fujisawa H, et al. Improvement of functional outcome after radical surgery in glioblastoma patients: the efficacy of a navigation-guided fence-post procedure and neurophysiological monitoring. J Neuro-Oncology. 2005;78(1):91–7. https://link.springer.com/article/10.1007/s11060-005-9064-2
7. Wu JS, Zhou LF, Tang WJ, Mao Y, Hu J, Song YY, et al. Clinical evaluation and follow-up outcome of diffusion tensor imaging-based functional neuronavigation: a prospective, controlled study in patients with gliomas involving pyramidal tracts. Neurosurgery. 2007;61(5):935–48.
8. Sherman JH, Hoes K, Marcus J, Komotar RJ, Brennan CW, Gutin PH. Neurosurgery for brain tumors: update on recent technical advances. Curr Neurol Neurosci Rep. 2011;11:313–219.
9. Kinoshita M, Tetsu AE, Ae G, Okita Y, Naoki AE, Ae K, et al. Diffusion tensor-based tumor infiltration index cannot discriminate vasogenic edema from tumor-infiltrated edema. J Neurooncol [Internet]. 2010;96:409–15. http://www.nf.mpg.de/vinci/
10. Janecek JK, Swanson SJ, Sabsevitz DS, Hammeke TA, Raghavan ME, Rozman M, et al. Language lateralization by fMRI and Wada testing in 229 patients with epilepsy: rates and predictors of discordance. Epilepsia [Internet]. 2013;54(2):314–22. https://onlinelibrary.wiley.com/doi/full/10.1111/epi.12068
11. Roux FE, Boulanouar K, Lotterie JA, Mejdoubi M, LeSage JP, Berry I, et al. Language functional magnetic resonance imaging in preoperative assessment of language areas: correlation with direct cortical stimulation. Neurosurgery [Internet]. 2003;52(6):1335–47. https://pubmed.ncbi.nlm.nih.gov/12762879/
12. Wehner T. The role of functional imaging in the tumor patient. Epilepsia [Internet]. 2013;54(Suppl 9):44–9. https://onlinelibrary.wiley.com/doi/full/10.1111/epi.12443
13. Giussani C, Roux FE, Ojemann J, Sganzerla EP, Pirillo D, Papagno C. Is preoperative functional magnetic resonance imaging reliable for language areas mapping in brain tumor surgery? Review of language functional magnetic resonance imaging and direct cortical stimulation correlation studies. Neurosurgery [Internet]. 2010;66(1):113–20. https://pubmed.ncbi.nlm.nih.gov/19935438/
14. Tate MC, Duffau H. Awake craniotomy and intraopertive mapping. In: Youmans and winn neurological surgery. 7th ed. 2017. p. 987–92.
15. Kubben PL, Cornips EM, Santbrink H van, Overbeeke JJ van. Intraoperative magnetic resonance imaging. In: Youmans and Winn neurological surgery. 7th ed. Elsevier; 2017. p. 2130–5.
16. Moiyadi AV, Shetty P, John R. Non-enhancing gliomas: does intraoperative ultrasonography improve resections? Ultrasonography [Internet]. 2018;38(2):156–65. http://www.e--ultrasonography.org/journal/view.php?doi=10.14366/usg.18032
17. Prada F, Solbiati L, Martegani A, DiMeco F. Intraoperative ultrasound (IOUS) in neurosurgery: from standard B-mode to elastosonography. 1st ed. Springer; 2016.
18. Unsgaard G, Rygh OM, Selbekk T, Müller TB, Kolstad F, Lindseth F, et al. Intra-operative 3D ultrasound in neurosurgery. Acta Neurochir (Wien) [Internet]. 2006;148(3):235–53. https://pubmed.ncbi.nlm.nih.gov/16362178/
19. Lindseth F, Langø T, Bang J, Hernes TAN. Accuracy evaluation of a 3D ultrasound-based neuronavigation system. Comput Aided Surg [Internet]. 2002;7(4):197–222. https://pubmed.ncbi.nlm.nih.gov/12454892/
20. Moiyadi AV, Kannan S, Shetty P. Navigated intraoperative ultrasound for resection of gliomas: predictive value, influence on resection and survival. Neurol India [Internet]. 2015;63(5):727. https://www.neurologyindia.com/article.asp?issn=0028-3886;year=2015;volume=63;issue=5;spage=727;epage=735;aulast=Moiyadi
21. Moiyadi AV, Shetty P, Singh V. ITVT-05. Intraoperative Ultrasound Guidance Improves Resection In Gliomas—Results From A Single Centre Propensity Matched Comparative Cohort Analysis Of 2D Vs Navigated 3D Ultrasound In 500 Gliomas. Neuro Oncol [Internet]. 2021;23(Suppl 6):vi228–9. https://academic.oup.com/neuro-oncology/article/23/Supplement_6/vi228/6426712

22. Prada F, Perin A, Martegani A, Aiani L, Solbiati L, Lamperti M, et al. Intraoperative contrast-enhanced ultrasound for brain tumor surgery. Neurosurgery [Internet]. 2022;74(5):542–52. https://pubmed.ncbi.nlm.nih.gov/24598809/
23. Chômas JE, Dayton P, Alien J, Morgan K, Ferrara KW. Mechanisms of contrast agent destruction. IEEE Trans Ultrason Ferroelectr Freq Control [Internet]. 2001;48(1):232–48. https://pubmed.ncbi.nlm.nih.gov/11367791/
24. Selbekk T, Bang J, Unsgaard G. Strain processing of intraoperative ultrasound images of brain tumours: initial results. Ultrasound Med Biol [Internet]. 2005;31(1):45–51. https://pubmed.ncbi.nlm.nih.gov/15653230/
25. Prada F, Del Bene M, Rampini A, Mattei L, Casali C, Vetrano IG, et al. Intraoperative strain elastosonography in brain tumor surgery. Oper Neurosurg [Internet]. 2019;17(2):227–36. https://journals.lww.com/onsonline/Fulltext/2019/08000/Intraoperative_Strain_Elastosonography_in_Brain.13.aspx
26. Sun H, Roberts DW, Farid H, Wu Z, Hartov A, Paulsen KD. Cortical surface tracking using a stereoscopic operating microscope. Neurosurgery [Internet]. 2005;56(Suppl 1):86–97. https://pubmed.ncbi.nlm.nih.gov/15799796/
27. Bagga V, Bhattacharyya D. Robotics in neurosurgery. Ann R Coll Surg Engl [Internet]. 2018;100(Suppl 6):23. /pmc/articles/PMC5956573/
28. Schucht P, Moritz-Gasser S, Herbet G, Raabe A, Duffau H. Subcortical electrostimulation to identify network subserving motor control. Hum Brain Mapp [Internet]. 2013;34(11):3023–30. https://pubmed.ncbi.nlm.nih.gov/22711688/
29. Rech F, Herbet G, Moritz-Gasser S, Duffau H. Disruption of bimanual movement by unilateral subcortical electrostimulation. Hum Brain Mapp [Internet]. 2014;35(7):3439. /pmc/articles/PMC6869258/
30. Pathiyil RK, Moiyadi AV, Shetty P, Singh V, Velayutham P. Transopercular approach to resection of dominant hemisphere diffuse insular glioma using multimodal intraoperative strategy with awake mapping. Neurol India [Internet]. 2022;70(2):520. https://www.neurologyindia.com/article.asp?issn=0028-3886;year=2022;volume=70;issue=2;spage=520;epage=523;aulast=Pathiyil
31. Tate MC, Herbet G, Moritz-Gasser S, Tate JE, Duffau H. Probabilistic map of critical functional regions of the human cerebral cortex: Broca's area revisited. Brain [Internet]. 2014;137(Pt 10):2773–82. https://pubmed.ncbi.nlm.nih.gov/24970097/
32. Lucas TH, McKhann GM, Ojemann GA. Functional separation of languages in the bilingual brain: a comparison of electrical stimulation language mapping in 25 bilingual patients and 117 monolingual control patients. J Neurosurg [Internet]. 2004;101(3):449–57. https://pubmed.ncbi.nlm.nih.gov/15352603/
33. Duffau H. Surgery of insular gliomas. Prog Neurol Surg [Internet]. 2018;30:173–85. https://www.karger.com/Article/FullText/464393
34. Sloan TB, Jameson L, Janik D. Evoked potentials. In: Cottrell and Young's Neuroanesthesia. 5th ed. Mosby Elsevier; 2010. p. 115–30.
35. Picht T, Schmidt S, Brandt S, Frey D, Hannula H, Neuvonen T, et al. Preoperative functional mapping for rolandic brain tumor surgery: comparison of navigated transcranial magnetic stimulation to direct cortical stimulation. Neurosurgery [Internet]. 2011;69(3):581–8. https://pubmed.ncbi.nlm.nih.gov/21430587/
36. Paiva WS, Fonoff ET, Marcolin MA, Cabrera HN, Teixeira MJ. Cortical mapping with navigated transcranial magnetic stimulation in low-grade glioma surgery. Neuropsychiatr Dis Treat [Internet]. 2012;8:197–201. https://pubmed.ncbi.nlm.nih.gov/22665996/
37. Haddad AF, Young JS, Berger MS, Tarapore PE. Preoperative applications of navigated transcranial magnetic stimulation. Front Neurol. 2021;11:1950.
38. Stummer W, Pichlmeier U, Meinel T, Wiestler OD, Zanella F, Reulen HJ. Fluorescence-guided surgery with 5-aminolevulinic acid for resection of malignant glioma: a randomised controlled multicentre phase III trial. Lancet Oncol [Internet]. 2006;7(5):392–401. https://pubmed.ncbi.nlm.nih.gov/16648043/

86 R. K. Pathiyil

39. Schebesch KM, Brawanski A, Hohenberger MS, Höhne J. Fluorescein sodium-guided surgery of malignant brain tumors: history, current concepts, and future project. Turk Neurosurg [Internet]. 2016;26(2):185–94. https://pubmed.ncbi.nlm.nih.gov/26956810/
40. Ferraro N, Barbarite E, Albert TR, Berchmans E, Shah AH, Bregy A, et al. The role of 5-aminolevulinic acid in brain tumor surgery: a systematic review. Neurosurg Rev. 2016;39(4):545–55.
41. La Rocca G, Sabatino G, Menna G, Altieri R, Ius T, Marchese E, et al. 5-Aminolevulinic acid false positives in cerebral neuro-oncology: not all that is fluorescent is tumor. A case-based update and literature review. World Neurosurg [Internet]. 2020;137:187–93. https://pubmed.ncbi.nlm.nih.gov/32058110/
42. Stummer W, Stocker S, Wagner S, Stepp H, Fritsch C, Goetz C, et al. Intraoperative detection of malignant gliomas by 5-aminolevulinic acid-induced porphyrin fluorescence. Neurosurgery [Internet]. 1998;42(3):518–26. https://pubmed.ncbi.nlm.nih.gov/9526986/
43. Kaneko S, Suero Molina E, Ewelt C, Warneke N, Stummer W. Fluorescence-based measurement of real-time kinetics of Protoporphyrin IX after 5-aminolevulinic acid administration in human in situ malignant gliomas. Neurosurgery [Internet]. 2019;85(4):E739–46. https://pubmed.ncbi.nlm.nih.gov/31058995/
44. Acerbi F, Broggi M, Schebesch KM, Höhne J, Cavallo C, De Laurentis C, et al. Fluorescein-guided surgery for resection of high-grade gliomas: a multicentric prospective Phase II Study (FLUOGLIO). Clin Cancer Res [Internet]. 2018;24(1):52–61. https://pubmed.ncbi.nlm.nih.gov/29018053/
45. Shinoda J, Yano H, Yoshimura SI, Okumura A, Kaku Y, Iwama T, et al. Fluorescence-guided resection of glioblastoma multiforme by using high-dose fluorescein sodium. Technical note. J Neurosurg [Internet]. 2003;99(3):597–603. https://pubmed.ncbi.nlm.nih.gov/12959452/
46. Da Silv CE, Da Silva VD, Da Silva JLB. Convexity meningiomas enhanced by sodium fluorescein. Surg Neurol Int [Internet]. 2014;5:PMC3927087. /pmc/articles/PMC3927087/
47. Dilek O, Ihsan A, Tulay H. Anaphylactic reaction after fluorescein sodium administration during intracranial surgery. J Clin Neurosci [Internet]. 2011;18(3):430–1. https://pubmed.ncbi.nlm.nih.gov/21237654/
48. Tanahashi S, Iida H, Dohi S. An anaphylactoid reaction after administration of fluorescein sodium during neurosurgery. Anesth Analg [Internet]. 2006;103(2):503. https://pubmed.ncbi.nlm.nih.gov/16861458/

Chapter 7
Neuroradiology

Joe M Das

1. Which of the following features in an MRI scan does not help to differentiate a brain abscess from a glioblastoma?

   (a) Susceptibility Weighted Imaging
   (b) Deep Transfer Learning
   (c) Hand-crafted Radiomics
   (d) Contrast-enhanced MRI

   Answer: d

   - Cerebral abscesses on SWI—high-intensity line (granulation tissue) lies internal to the low-intensity rim—The dual rim sign

2. Which of the following is not a characterizing magnetic resonance spectroscopy finding in a glioblastoma?

   (a) Increased choline
   (b) Increased myoinositol
   (c) Increased lactate
   (d) Increased lipids

   Answer: b

J. M. Das (✉)
Consultant Neurosurgeon, Bahrain Specialist Hospital, Juffair, Bahrain
e-mail: neurosurgeon@doctors.org.uk

© The Author(s), under exclusive license to Springer Nature
Switzerland AG 2023
J. M. Das, *Neuro-Oncology Explained Through Multiple Choice Questions*,
https://doi.org/10.1007/978-3-031-13253-7_7

3. Match the following subtypes of medulloblastomas with the corresponding likely location or spectroscopy feature.

(a) WNT	Midline
(b) SHH	Cerebellar peduncle/foramen of Luschka
(c) Group 3 or 4	Cerebellar hemisphere
(c) SHH	Taurine peak
(d) Group 3 or 4	No taurine

Answer:

(a) WNT	Cerebellar peduncle/foramen of Luschka
(b) SHH	Cerebellar hemisphere
(c) Group 3 or 4	Midline
(c) SHH	No taurine
(d) Group 3 or 4	Taurine peak

4. What is the usual location of a posterior fossa type A ependymoma?

   (a) Apex of the fourth ventricle
   (b) Lateral recess of the fourth ventricle
   (c) The midline of the fourth ventricle near the obex
   (d) Superior medullary velum

   Answer: b

   - PFA Ependymoma—Lateral recess of the fourth ventricle
   - PFB Ependymoma—Midline of the fourth ventricle near the obex

5. Match the following radiological signs with the corresponding tumors.

(a) Periwinkle sign	Brain stem glioma
(b) Yin-yang sign	Primary CNS lymphoma
(c) Notch sign	Solitary fibrous tumor of the dura
(d) Spoke wheel sign	Meningioma
(e) Mother-in-law sign on angiography	Leptomeningeal carcinomatosis
(f) Pool sign	Supratentorial ependymoma
(g) Flat floor of fourth ventricle sign	Metastatic adenocarcinoma
(h) Bright rim sign	Dyembryoplastic neuroepithelial tumor
(i) T2-FLAIR mismatch sign	Vestibular schwannoma
(j) Trumpeted internal acoustic meatus sign	Meningioma
(k) Snowman sign	Meningioma
(l) Volcano sign	Diffuse astrocytoma
(m) Sugar coating sign	Pituitary macroadenoma

Answer:

(a) Periwinkle sign	Supratentorial ependymoma
(b) Yin-yang sign	Solitary fibrous tumor of the dura
(c) Notch sign	Primary CNS lymphoma
(d) Spoke wheel sign	Meningioma

(e) Mother-in-law sign on angiography	Meningioma
(f) Pool sign	Metastatic adenocarcinoma
(g) Flat floor of fourth ventricle sign	Brain stem glioma
(h) Bright rim sign	Dysembryoplastic neuroepithelial tumor
(i) T2-FLAIR mismatch sign	Diffuse astrocytoma
(j) Trumpeted internal acoustic meatus sign	Vestibular schwannoma
(k) Snowman sign	Pituitary macroadenoma
(l) Volcano sign	Meningioma
(m) Sugar coating sign	Leptomeningeal carcinomatosis

6. Match the following terms with their corresponding explanations.

(a) Artificial intelligence	Combines quantitative data from medical images with genomic phenotypes and creates a prediction model
(b) Machine learning	Feed-forward networks used for image-based problems
(c) Deep learning	Learning based on neural networks that have a large number of layers
(d) Convolutional neural networks	A task performed by a computer that normally needs human intelligence
(e) Radiomics	Method for quantitative description of medical images
(f) Delta-radiomics	Use of an individual's genetic profile to guide prevention, diagnosis, and treatment of diseases
(g) Radiogenomics	Changes in radiomic features from one point in time to the next
(h) Personalised medicine	A branch of data science which makes computers capable of learning from existing training data without accurate programming

Answer:

(a) Artificial intelligence	A task performed by a computer that normally needs human intelligence
(b) Machine learning	A branch of data science which makes computers capable of learning from existing training data without accurate programming
(c) Deep learning	Learning based on neural networks that have a large number of layers
(d) Convolutional neural networks	Feed-forward networks used for image-based problems
(e) Radiomics	Method for quantitative description of medical images
(f) Delta-radiomics	Changes in radiomic features from one point in time to the next
(g) Radiogenomics	Combines quantitative data from medical images with genomic phenotypes and creates a prediction model
(h) Personalised medicine	Use of an individual's genetic profile to guide prevention, diagnosis, and treatment of diseases.

7. The term "pseudoprogression" refers to the occurrence of a progressively enhancing lesion on magnetic resonance imaging scan within what duration of radiotherapy?

   (a) 4 weeks
   (b) 8 weeks
   (c) 12 weeks
   (d) 24 weeks

   Answer: c

8. Which of the following is a characteristic feature present in vasogenic tumoral edema that differentiates it from cytotoxic edema on imaging?

   (a) Violates the boundary at gray matter-white matter junction
   (b) Does not violate the boundary at gray matter-white matter junction
   (c) Follows a circular pattern
   (d) Follows an oval pattern

   Answer: b

Cytotoxic edema affects predominantly the gray matter causing a loss of gray-white differentiation.

9. Match the following tumors with their peculiar metabolites on magnetic resonance imaging:

(a) PNET	GLX (Glutamate, Glutamine, GABA)
(b) Meningioma	Alanine
(c) Glioblastoma	Myoinositol
(d) Low-grade astrocytomas	Taurine
(e) Oligodendroglioma, demyelination	Glycine

   Answer:

(a) PNET	Taurine
(b) Meningioma	Alanine
(c) Glioblastoma	Glycine
(d) Low-grade astrocytomas	Myoinositol
(e) Oligodendroglioma, demyelination	GLX (Glutamate, Glutamine, GABA)

10. Which of the following is used as the internal reference standard for characterizing other peaks during MRS?

    (a) Choline
    (b) Creatinine
    (c) NAA
    (d) Lactate

    Answer: b

11. Gallium-68 DOTATATE PET scan is useful in the characterization of

    (a) High-grade glioma
    (b) Low-grade glioma
    (c) Metastases
    (d) Meningioma

    Answer: d

12. Which tumor is not a part of the MISME syndrome?

    (a) Schwannoma
    (b) Meningioma
    (c) Ependymoma
    (d) Medulloblastoma

    Answer: d

    MISME—Multiple   Inherited   Schwannomas,   Meningiomas,   and
    Ependymomas.

13. Which of the following is not a criterion to be met for a positive "dural tail" sign?

    (a) The tail should be seen on two consecutive images through the tumor
    (b) The tail should taper away from the tumor
    (c) The tail should enhance more than the tumor
    (d) The tail should be shorter than half the diameter of the tumor

    Answer: d

14. The tram-track sign on contrast-enhanced CT/MRI helps differentiate which of the following conditions?

    (a) Tuberculum sellae and suprasellar meningioma
    (b) Cerebellopontine angle schwannoma and meningioma
    (c) Optic nerve sheath meningioma and glioma
    (d) Falx meningioma from petroclival meningioma

    Answer: c

    • Tram-track sign—Two enhancing areas of tumor separated by the negative defect due to optic nerve.
    • Classically seen in optic nerve sheath meningioma and absent in optic glioma.
    • Also seen in orbital pseudotumor, perioptic neuritis, sarcoidosis, and lymphomas.

15. The "bare orbit" sign is seen in which condition?

    (a) Orbital pseudotumor
    (b) Neurofibromatosis 1
    (c) Orbital lymphangioma
    (d) Orbital hemangioma

    Answer: b

Bare orbit sign:

- Seen in a frontal radiograph
- Absence of innominate line (projection of greater wing of sphenoid)
- Seen in sphenoid wing dysplasia—neurofibromatosis 1

16. Radial bands sign is seen in

    (a) Neurofibromatosis 1
    (b) Neurofibromatosis 2
    (c) Tuberous sclerosis
    (d) Von Hippel-Lindau syndrome

    Answer: c

    Radial bands sign:

    - Linear signal intensities from periventricular to subcortical regions in FLAIR sequences.
    - Seen in tuberous sclerosis (also known as Bourneville disease or Bourneville-Pringle disease)
    - Abnormal migration of dysplastic stem cells.

17. Match the following imaging techniques with the information they provide.

(a) Amide proton transfer imaging	Separation of perfusion from diffusion
(b) Contrast-enhanced susceptibility-weighted imaging	Tumor vascular normalization and drug delivery efficacy
(c) Arterial spin labeling	Tumor proliferation and provides information regarding the pH of tissue
(d) Dynamic contrast-enhanced perfusion MRI	Tumor necrosis and vessels.
(e) Dynamic susceptibility contrast perfusion MRI	Estimation of cytoarchitectonic complexities of gray and white matters
(f) Diffusion Kurtosis Imaging (DKI)	Microvessel density or area
(g) Intravoxel Incoherent Motion (IVIM)	Identification of immature hyperpermeable vessels

    Answer:

(a) Amide proton transfer imaging	Tumor proliferation and provides information regarding the pH of tissue
(b) Contrast-enhanced susceptibility-weighted imaging	Tumor necrosis and vessels.
(c) Arterial spin labeling	Tumor vascular normalization and drug delivery efficacy
(d) Dynamic contrast-enhanced perfusion MRI	Identification of immature hyperpermeable vessels.
(e) Dynamic susceptibility contrast perfusion MRI	Microvessel density or area
(f) Diffusion Kurtosis Imaging (DKI)	Estimation of cytoarchitectonic complexities of gray and white matters
(g) Intravoxel Incoherent Motion (IVIM)	Separation of perfusion from diffusion

Test your learning and check your understanding of this book's contents: use the "Springer Nature Flashcards" app to access questions using https://sn.pub/3HwHCw To use the app, please follow the instructions in Chap. 1.

Bibliography

1. Bo L, Zhang Z, Jiang Z, Yang C, Huang P, Chen T, Wang Y, Yu G, Tan X, Cheng Q, Li D, Liu Z. Differentiation of brain abscess from cystic glioma using conventional MRI based on deep transfer learning features and hand-crafted radiomics features. Front Med (Lausanne). 2021;8:748144. https://doi.org/10.3389/fmed.2021.748144.
2. Rudie JD, Rauschecker AM, Bryan RN, Davatzikos C, Mohan S. Emerging applications of artificial intelligence in neuro-oncology. Radiology. 2019;290(3):607–18. https://doi.org/10.1148/radiol.2018181928. Epub 2019 Jan 22
3. van Timmeren JE, Cester D, Tanadini-Lang S, Alkadhi H, Baessler B. Radiomics in medical imaging-"how-to" guide and critical reflection. Insights Imaging. 2020;11(1):91. https://doi.org/10.1186/s13244-020-00887-2.
4. Lo Gullo R, Daimiel I, Morris EA, Pinker K. Combining molecular and imaging metrics in cancer: radiogenomics. Insights Imaging. 2020;11(1):1. https://doi.org/10.1186/s13244-019-0795-6.
5. www.genome.gov
6. Kocher M, Ruge MI, Galldiks N, Lohmann P. Applications of radiomics and machine learning for radiotherapy of malignant brain tumors. Strahlenther Onkol. 2020;196(10):856–67. https://doi.org/10.1007/s00066-020-01626-8. Epub 2020 May 11
7. Jha SK. Cerebral edema and its management. Med J Armed Forces India. 2003;59(4):326–31. https://doi.org/10.1016/S0377-1237(03)80147-8. Epub 2011 Jul 21
8. Verma A, Kumar I, Verma N, Aggarwal P, Ojha R. Magnetic resonance spectroscopy—revisiting the biochemical and molecular milieu of brain tumors. BBA Clin. 2016;5:170–8. https://doi.org/10.1016/j.bbacli.2016.04.002.
9. Ivanidze J, Roytman M, Lin E, Magge RS, Pisapia DJ, Liechty B, Karakatsanis N, Ramakrishna R, Knisely J, Schwartz TH, Osborne JR, Pannullo SC. Gallium-68 DOTATATE PET in the evaluation of intracranial meningiomas. J Neuroimaging. 2019;29(5):650–6. https://doi.org/10.1111/jon.12632.
10. Gupta A, Gupta C, Sachan M, Singh S. Extensive cranial nerves involvement in Neurofibromatosis: a rare presentation. J Pediatr Neurosci. 2018;13(1):74–7. https://doi.org/10.4103/JPN.JPN_32_18.
11. Chavhan GB, Shroff MM. Twenty classic signs in neuroradiology: a pictorial essay. Indian J Radiol Imaging. 2009;19(2):135–45. https://doi.org/10.4103/0971-3026.50835.
12. Kim M, Kim HS. Emerging techniques in brain tumor imaging: what radiologists need to know. Korean J Radiol. 2016;17(5):598–619. https://doi.org/10.3348/kjr.2016.17.5.598.

Chapter 8
Chemotherapy

Ebtesam Abdulla, Luis Rafael Moscote-Salazar, Amit Agrawal, and Daulat Singh

1. You are evaluating a 28-year-old man with a known history of HIV infection who presented with persistent headaches. Imaging demonstrated a classic appearance of primary CNS lymphoma. What is the best initial treatment for these lesions?

   (a) Observation
   (b) Gross total resection
   (c) Chemotherapy with methotrexate
   (d) Chemotherapy with Hydroxyurea

   Answer: c

   Primary CNS lymphoma is highly radiosensitive and methotrexate-sensitive. Methotrexate is the most effective first therapy. Gross complete resection is contraindicated because of the substantial postoperative morbidity. Hydroxyurea is used to treat meningiomas [1].

E. Abdulla (✉)
Department of Neurosurgery, Salmaniya Medical Complex, Manama, Bahrain
e-mail: EQooti@health.gov.bh

L. R. Moscote-Salazar
Colombian Clinical Research Group in Neurocritical Care, Bogota, Colombia

A. Agrawal
Department of Neurosurgery, All India Institute of Medical Sciences,
Bhopal, Madhya Pradesh, India

D. Singh
Department of Radiation Oncology, Govt Doon Medical College & Hospital,
Dehradun, Uttarakhand, India

J. M. Das, *Neuro-Oncology Explained Through Multiple Choice Questions*,
https://doi.org/10.1007/978-3-031-13253-7_8

2. A tumor was resected from a 61-year-old man with convulsions. The pathological evaluation of the specimen was consistent with WHO grade 4 glioblastoma multiforme (GBM). A chemotherapeutic temozolomide was commenced. What is the most common side effect of temozolomide?

(a) Renal toxicity
(b) Liver toxicity
(c) Keratitis
(d) Bone marrow suppression

Answer: d

Temozolomide is a chemotherapeutic agent that is well tolerated. It may nevertheless cause thrombocytopenia and neutropenia. Temozolomide has also been associated with severe hematologic side effects, including myelodysplastic syndrome and aplastic anemia [2].

3. What tumor type listed below is most likely to respond to the ICE regimen (ifosfamide, carboplatin, etoposide)?

(a) Germ cells tumors
(b) Medulloblastoma
(c) Glioblastoma multiforme
(d) Primary CNS lymphoma

Answer: a

Two cycles of the ICE regimen, which consists of ifosfamide ($2 \ gm/m^2$), carboplatin ($400 \ mg/m^2$), and etoposide ($20 \ mg/m^2$), followed by autologous hematopoietic progenitor cell support, is a potential treatment for germ cell malignancies [3].

4. Which one of the following chemotherapy options is LEAST likely to be utilized in the context of anaplastic oligodendroglioma?

(a) Procarbazine
(b) Lomustine
(c) Etoposide
(d) Vincristine

Answer: c

It is possible to treat anaplastic oligodendroglioma with a combination of radiation therapy, chemotherapy, and surgery. For the treatment of low-grade glioma, studies have mostly focused on the three-drug combination of procarbazine, lomustine, and vincristine (PCV) or a single dosage of temozolomide [4].

5. Which one of the following statements regarding vinca alkaloids is LEAST accurate?

(a) They prevent tubulin polymerization and thus microtubule formation
(b) Induce cell apoptosis by arresting growing cells in the S phase.

(c) Peripheral neuropathy is a possible side effect
(d) Vincristine is an example of a first-generation agent.

Answer: b

Vinca alkaloids, which belong to a family of cell cycle phase M-specific anti-tubulin medicines, were among the first plant alkaloids identified for use in humans as anti-cancer drugs. *Vinca rosea* (*Catharanthus roseus*) alkaloids include first-generation (vincristine, vinblastine), second-generation semisynthetic derivatives (vinorelbine, vindesine), and third-generation alkaloids (vinflunine). Some have also classed vinflunine as a second-generation agent [5].

6. Which one of the following chemotherapy options is used for subependymal giant cell astrocytoma (SEGA)?

(a) Everolimus
(b) Methotrexate
(c) Vincristine
(d) Erlotinib

Answer: a

Over 5 years of therapy, everolimus continues to have a sustained impact on SEGA tumor regression. It was determined that Everolimus was well tolerated and that no new safety concerns had arisen [6].

7. Which one of the following chemotherapy options is a vascular endothelial growth factor (VEGF) inhibitor?

(a) Carmustine
(b) Tamoxifen
(c) Everolimus
(d) Bevacizumab

Answer: d

Bevacizumab (Avastin®), a VEGF inhibitor, has been utilized as a salvage treatment for patients with recurrent GBM in the United States since 2009 [7].

8. You are monitoring a 19-year-old man with medulloblastoma for which surgery was done. Concurrent chemotherapy was started. The patient developed hearing loss. Which chemotherapeutic agent was used?

(a) mTOR inhibitor
(b) Alkylating agent
(c) Dihydrofolate reductase inhibitor
(d) Platinum alkylating agent

Answer: d

Widely used to treat medulloblastoma, cisplatin is a very efficient chemotherapeutic drug. However, its usage has been linked to substantial adverse effects, including bilateral, gradual, irreversible, dose-dependent neurosensory hearing loss [8].

9. Which of the following chemotherapeutic option is used as a wafer for GBM?

 (a) Cisplatin
 (b) Lomustine
 (c) Temozolomide
 (d) Carmustine

Answer: d

Carmustine wafers show potential as an effective therapy for GBM patients compared to alternative treatment options. Carmustine wafers should be studied further in bigger randomized controlled trials for the treatment of GBM patients as a monotherapy or combo therapy [9].

10. What metabolic derangement does chemotherapy lead to?

 (a) Hypercalcemia
 (b) Hypokalemia
 (c) Hypocalcemia
 (d) Hypophosphatemia

Answer: c

Acute renal failure and severe electrolyte imbalances are common symptoms of tumor lysis syndrome, an oncologic emergency. The condition often manifests in individuals with lymphoproliferative cancers, typically after the commencement of chemotherapy. Hyperkalemia, hyperphosphatemia, hyperuricemia, and hypocalcemia are defining characteristics [10].

11. The final pathology of a tumor resected from a 42-year-old woman's brain is mixed oligoastrocytoma. The patient started on the PCV regimen. What dietary to AVOID while on the PCV regimen?

 (a) Sugar-containing food
 (b) Tyramine-containing food
 (c) Iodine-containing food
 (d) Estrogen-rich food

Answer: b

When taken with tyramine-containing meals, procarbazine, an alkylating medication, causes malignant hypertension in the patient [11].

12. Concerning the delivery of chemotherapy to the brain, which of the following is LEAST likely to contribute to the low permeability of the blood-brain barrier (BBB)?

 (a) Increased pinocytic activity reflecting a low level of transcellular transport
 (b) Interaction of astrocytic processes and pericytes with brain endothelial cells

(c) Presence of ATP-binding cassette transporters

(d) Presence of insulin receptors

Answer: a

Between the blood and the brain lies a barrier known as the blood-brain barrier (BBB), which is a highly selective barrier. The low pinocytic activity reflects a low level of transcellular transport, the interaction of astrocytic processes and pericytes with brain endothelial cells, presence of ATP-binding cassette transporters, insulin receptors, multidrug resistance–associated proteins, and transferrin receptors, lack of lymphatic drainage, and absence of major histocompatibility complex all contribute to the low permeability of the BBB [12].

13. Which of the following brain tumors is NOT typically treated with chemotherapy?

(a) Chordoma

(b) Ependymoma

(c) Meningioma

(d) Astrocytoma

Answer: b

Following astrocytoma and medulloblastoma, ependymoma is the third most frequent pediatric brain tumor, with an estimated 200 new occurrences each year. The importance of neurosurgeons in the treatment of ependymomas in children is highlighted by the high probability of cure for patients who have an extensive complete resection. The standard of treatment is complete gross resection followed by radiation. Typically, chemotherapy is not part of the treatment protocol [13].

14. You are asked to evaluate an NF1 child with optic pathway glioma (OPG) depicted in the MRI. The patient presented with progressive visual decline, and severe exophthalmos. What is the best initial treatment for this condition?

(a) Chemotherapy plus radiotherapy

(b) Surgery

(c) Observation

(d) Chemotherapy alone

Answer: d

Chemotherapy is the cornerstone of treatment, with most regimens consisting of carboplatin and vincristine. The five-year survival rate exceeds 90 percent with chemotherapy alone and may significantly delay or postpone radiation treatment for children with OPG. Surgical intervention may be considered if eyesight has been lost. Radiation treatment for NF1 poses a substantial risk of subsequent malignancy, cognitive impairment, and vascular stenosis, and should be undertaken with caution [14].

15. You are evaluating a patient with a recurrent systemic Langerhans Cell Histiocytosis involving the CNS. What targeted gene therapy is likely effective in this patient?

    (a) VEGF inhibitor
    (b) BRAF inhibitor
    (c) PTEN inhibitor
    (d) P53 inhibitor

    Answer: b

    Surgery is the treatment for Langerhans Cell Histiocytosis. Persistence or recurrence of these lesions, however, may demand further treatment, such as low-dose chemotherapy or, in rare instances, low-dose radiation therapy. The findings of targeted treatment with BRAF inhibitors for systemic illness are promising [15].

16. What is the best management of a patient with a biopsy-proven, non-AIDS-related primary CNS lymphoma?

    (a) Surgical resection followed by XRT
    (b) Surgical resection followed by methotrexate chemotherapy
    (c) Surgical resection followed by XRT and methotrexate chemotherapy
    (d) XRT and methotrexate chemotherapy

    Answer: d

    The most effective treatment for primary CNS lymphoma in patients without AIDS is a combination of X-ray radiotherapy and methotrexate chemotherapy. There is no justification for surgical excision [16].

17. What is the best management of a patient with biopsy-proven, metastatic non-small-cell lung cancer?

    (a) Erlotinib
    (b) Avastin
    (c) Methotrexate
    (d) Vincristine

    Answer: a

    Erlotinib is an oral tyrosine kinase inhibitor that targets the human epidermal receptor type 1/ epidermal growth factor receptor. It was recently authorized by the FDA for the treatment of patients with locally advanced or metastatic non-small-cell lung cancer who have failed more than one or two previous chemotherapy regimens [17].

18. What is the following chemotherapy agent contributing to delayed wound healing?

    (a) Erlotinib
    (b) Avastin®

(c) Tamoxifen
(d) Methotrexate

Answer: b

Using Avastin® may result in bleeding or infection as a consequence of wounds not healing properly. The patient must discontinue bevacizumab at least 28 days before undergoing any form of surgery. After surgery, Avastin® should not be resumed for at least 28 days, or until the surgical incision has healed [18].

19. You are evaluating a 60-year-old patient, known to have colorectal cancer, and recently diagnosed with GBM. Which of the following concerns of starting bevacizumab in this case?

(a) Megacolon
(b) Bowel perforation
(c) Liver metastasis
(d) Mesenteric venous thrombosis

Answer: b

The majority of bowel perforations caused by Avastin® (bevacizumab) have occurred when the tumor penetrates the colon's wall. Avastin® causes the tumor to disintegrate, leaving behind a void. With Avastin®, the tumor disappears, but scar tissue does not develop since the tumor is unable to generate its blood supply [19].

20. You are evaluating a patient with brain lymphoma who developed generalized tonic-clonic convulsions after intrathecal injection. Which of the following chemotherapeutic agent was likely given?

(a) Lomustine
(b) Vincristine
(c) Cisplatin
(d) Methotrexate

Answer: d

The intrathecal injection of methotrexate may achieve therapeutic concentrations in the cerebrospinal fluid without the use of intravenous methotrexate at large doses. 3-to-40 percent of individuals receiving intrathecal methotrexate have been documented to have major neurologic problems. Dosage, methotrexate concentration in CSF, patient age, anatomical and physiological abnormalities in the CNS, type of dilutional vehicle, intracranial radiation, and intravenous methotrexate are all factors that contribute to the development of neurotoxicity [20].

Test your learning and check your understanding of this book's contents: use the "Springer Nature Flashcards" app to access questions using https://sn.pub/3HwHCw To use the app, please follow the instructions in Chap. 1.

Bibliography

1. Bernstein B. Neuro-oncology: the essentials. 3rd ed. Thieme; 2015. p. 439–48.
2. Scaringi C, De Sanctis V, Minniti G, et al. Temozolomide-related hematologic toxicity. Onkologie. 2013;36(7–8):444–9.
3. Lotz JP, André T, Bouleuc C, et al. The ICE regimen (ifosfamide, carboplatin, etoposide) for the treatment of germ-cell tumors and metastatic trophoblastic disease. Bone Marrow Transplant. 1996;18(Suppl 1):S55–9.
4. Webre C, Shonka N, Smith L, et al. PC or PCV, that is the question: primary anaplastic Oligodendroglial tumors treated with Procarbazine and CCNU with and without vincristine. Anticancer Res. 2015;35(10):5467–72.
5. Loh K. Know the medicinal herb: Catharanthus roseus (Vinca rosea). Malays Fam Physician. 2008;3(2):123.
6. Franz DN, Agricola K, Mays M, et al. Everolimus for subependymal giant cell astrocytoma: 5-year final analysis. Ann Neurol. 2015;78(6):929–38.
7. Kreisl TN, Kim L, Moore K, et al. Phase II trial of single-agent bevacizumab followed by bevacizumab plus irinotecan at tumor progression in recurrent glioblastoma. J Clin Oncol. 2009;27(5):740–5.
8. Callejo A, Sedó-Cabezón L, Juan ID, Llorens J. Cisplatin-Induced ototoxicity: effects, mechanisms and protection strategies. Toxics. 2015;3(3):268–93.
9. Zhang YD, Dai RY, Chen Z, et al. Efficacy and safety of carmustine wafers in the treatment of glioblastoma multiforme: a systematic review. Turk Neurosurg. 2014;24(5):639–45.
10. Davidson MB, Thakkar S, Hix JK, et al. Pathophysiology, clinical consequences, and treatment of tumor lysis syndrome. Am J Med. 2004;116(8):546–54.
11. Collado-Borrell R, Escudero-Vilaplana V, Romero-Jiménez R, Iglesias-Peinado I, Herranz-Alonso A, Sanjurjo-Sáez M. Oral antineoplastic agent interactions with medicinal plants and food: an issue to take into account. J Cancer Res Clin Oncol. 2016;142(11):2319–30.
12. Zou L, Ma JL, Wang T, et al. Cell-penetrating peptide-mediated therapeutic molecule delivery into the central nervous system. Curr Neuropharmacol. 2013;11:197–208.
13. McGuire CS, Sainani KL, Fisher PG. Incidence patterns for ependymoma: a surveillance, epidemiology, and end results study. J Neurosurg. 2009;110(4):725–9.
14. Laithier V, Grill J, Le Deley MC, et al. Progression-free survival in children with optic pathway tumors: dependence on age and the quality of the response to chemotherapy--results of the first French prospective study for the French Society of Pediatric Oncology. J Clin Oncol. 2003;21(24):4572–8.
15. Grana N. Langerhans cell histiocytosis. Cancer Control. 2014;21(4):328–34.
16. Batchelor T, Carson K, O'Neill A, et al. Treatment of primary CNS lymphoma with methotrexate and deferred radiotherapy: a report of NABTT 96-07. J Clin Oncol. 2003;21(6):1044–9.
17. Smith J. Erlotinib: small-molecule targeted therapy in the treatment of non-small-cell lung cancer. Clin Ther. 2005;27(10):1513–34.
18. Zhang H, Huang Z, Zou X, Liu T. Bevacizumab and wound-healing complications: a systematic review and meta-analysis of randomized controlled trials. Oncotarget. 2016;7(50):82473–81.
19. Heinzerling JH, Huerta S. Bowel perforation from bevacizumab for the treatment of metastatic colon cancer: incidence, etiology, and management. Curr Surg. 2006;63(5):334–7.
20. Pui CH, Howard SC. Current management and challenges of malignant disease in the CNS in paediatric leukaemia. Lancet Oncol. 2008;9:257–68.

Chapter 9
Radiotherapy

Joe M Das

1. Which of the following medicines has been tried to ameliorate the neurocognitive effects of whole-brain radiotherapy?

   (a) Trastuzumab
   (b) Folic acid
   (c) Memantine
   (d) Folinic acid

   Answer: c

   Memantine—N- methyl-D-aspartate-receptor antagonist

2. Match the following side effects to the period when they occur following radiation therapy.

(a) Radiation-induced seizures	Days to weeks
(b) Cerebral edema	1-6 months
(c) Radiation necrosis	1-6 months
(b) Alopecia	Days to weeks
(e) Neuropraxia	Days to weeks
(f) Somnolence syndrome	6-24 months

   Answer:

(a) Radiation-induced seizures	Days to weeks
(b) Cerebral edema	Days to weeks
(c) Radiation necrosis	6–24 months
(b) Alopecia	Days to weeks
(e) Neuropraxia	1–6 months
(f) Somnolence syndrome	1–6 months

J. M. Das (✉)
Consultant Neurosurgeon, Bahrain Specialist Hospital, Juffair, Bahrain
e-mail: neurosurgeon@doctors.org.uk

© The Author(s), under exclusive license to Springer Nature
Switzerland AG 2023
J. M. Das, *Neuro-Oncology Explained Through Multiple Choice Questions*,
https://doi.org/10.1007/978-3-031-13253-7_9

3. Which part of the brain is spared during intensity-modulated radiotherapy in an attempt to reduce cognitive decline?

    (a) Periventricular stem cells
    (b) Dorsal medulla
    (c) Ventral medulla
    (d) Hippocampal neural stem cells

    Answer: d

4. What is the current standard of care for glioblastoma after tumor debulking surgery?

    (a) Radiation (60 Gy in 30 fractions) + Temozolomide followed by Temozolomide alone for 6 months
    (b) Radiation (60 Gy in 30 fractions) followed by Temozolomide alone for 6 months
    (c) Radiation (60 Gy in 60 fractions) + Temozolomide followed by Temozolomide alone for 12 months
    (d) Radiation (30 Gy in 60 fractions) followed by Temozolomide alone for 6 months

    Answer: a

5. Which of the following is a biomarker to predict the outcome and subsequent increased risk of radiotherapy before starting irradiation?

    (a) Micronuclei
    (b) TGF-β
    (c) FGF-2
    (d) Ang-1

    Answer: a

    • Predictive biomarkers: IL-1, IL-6, micronuclei
    • Prognostic biomarkers: TGF-β, FGF-2

6. Tumour-treating fields (TTFields) treatment should be administered continuously, for at least how many hours per day?

    (a) 6 h
    (b) 12 h
    (c) 18 h
    (d) 24 h

    Answer: c

    • TTFields are nonionizing
    • Delivered at an intermediate frequency (200 kHz for GBM) and low intensities (1–3 V/cm)

7. What is the most common device-related adverse event reported with TTFields treatment?

    (a) Seizures
    (b) Skin toxicity
    (c) Infection
    (d) Insomnia

    Answer: b

8. Which of the following is not an unfavorable prognostic factor for survival in a patient with low-grade glioma according to the European Organisation for Research and Treatment of Cancer Trials (EORTC)?

    (a) Age less than 40 years
    (b) Astrocytoma histology
    (c) Tumor diameter more than 6 cm
    (d) Tumor crossing midline

    Answer: a

    High-risk features in patients with low-grade glioma:

    - Age 40 or older
    - Astrocytoma histology
    - Tumor diameter $\geq$ 6 cm
    - Tumor crossing the midline
    - The presence of neurologic deficit before surgery

9. Which of the following is not included in the 4Rs involved in the radiobiology of ionizing radiation?

    (a) Repair
    (b) Regeneration
    (c) Repopulation
    (d) Reoxygenation

    Answer: b

    The biological effect of ionizing radiation to a given tissue is determined by:

    - Repair capacity of cells
    - Repopulation of surviving tumor stem cells
    - Redistribution of cells between the cell cycle
    - Reoxygenation of hypoxic tumor cells

10. Which part of the brain is most radioresistant?

    (a) Frontal lobe
    (b) Parietal lobe
    (c) Temporal lobe
    (d) Cerebellum

    Answer: a

- The radiosensitivity increases in the following order:

  Frontal region < parietal region < temporal lobe < cerebellar and brainstem < thalamus/basal ganglia.

11. Which drug has shown some promise in treating post-radiation cognitive symptoms?

    (a) Galantamine
    (b) Rivastigmine
    (c) Donepezil
    (d) Aducanumab

    Answer: c

12. Mitotically active neural stem cells are located within which part of the hippocampus?

    (a) Subpyramidal zone of the dentate gyrus
    (b) Subgranular zone of the dentate gyrus
    (c) Subpyramidal zone of the hippocampal gyrus
    (d) Subgranular zone of the hippocampal gyrus

    Answer: b

13. The maximum dose of radiation that can be given over the optic chiasm via stereotactic radiosurgery as per Quantitative Analysis of Normal Tissue Effects in the Clinic (QUANTEC) is

    (a) 2 Gy
    (b) 4 Gy
    (c) 6 Gy
    (d) 8 Gy

    Answer: d

    - Brainstem—maximum radiation—54 Gy; with SRS—12.5 Gy
    - Cochlea—12-14 Gy

14. Which hormone is most susceptible to irradiation among the hypothalamic-pituitary hormones?

    (a) Prolactin
    (b) Growth hormone
    (c) Adrenocorticotrophic hormone
    (d) Thyroid stimulating hormone

    Answer: b

15. Which pediatric brain tumor is most commonly treated with proton therapy?

    (a) Medulloblastoma
    (b) Atypical teratoid rhabdoid tumor
    (c) Brainstem glioma
    (d) Craniopharyngioma

    Answer: a

Test your learning and check your understanding of this book's contents: use the "Springer Nature Flashcards" app to access questions using https://sn.pub/3HwHCw To use the app, please follow the instructions in Chap. 1.

Bibliography

1. Lynch M. Preservation of cognitive function following whole brain radiotherapy in patients with brain metastases: complications, treatments, and the emerging role of memantine. J Oncol Pharm Pract. 2019;25(3):657–62. https://doi.org/10.1177/1078155218798176. Epub 2018 Sep 10
2. Wujanto C, Vellayappan B, Chang EL, Chao ST, Sahgal A, Lo SS. Radiotherapy to the brain: what are the consequences of this age-old treatment? Ann Palliat Med. 2021;10(1):936–52. Epub 2020 Jul 29
3. Barani IJ, Larson DA. Radiation therapy of glioblastoma. Cancer Treat Res. 2015;163:49–73. https://doi.org/10.1007/978-3-319-12048-5_4.
4. Sultana N, Sun C, Katsube T, Wang B. Biomarkers of brain damage induced by radiotherapy. Dose Response. 2020;18(3):1559325820938279. https://doi.org/10.1177/1559325820938279.
5. Trusheim J, Dunbar E, Battiste J, Iwamoto F, Mohile N, Damek D, Bota DA, Connelly J. A state-of-the-art review and guidelines for tumor treating fields treatment planning and patient follow-up in glioblastoma. CNS Oncol. 2017;6(1):29–43. https://doi.org/10.2217/cns-2016-0032. Epub 2016 Sep 15
6. Pignatti F, van den Bent M, Curran D, Debruyne C, Sylvester R, Therasse P, Afra D, Cornu P, Bolla M, Vecht C, Karim AB, European Organization for Research and Treatment of Cancer Brain Tumor Cooperative Group. European Organization for Research and Treatment of cancer radiotherapy cooperative group. Prognostic factors for survival in adult patients with cerebral low-grade glioma. J Clin Oncol. 2002;20(8):2076–84. https://doi.org/10.1200/JCO.2002.08.121.
7. Pajonk F, Vlashi E, McBride WH. Radiation resistance of cancer stem cells: the 4 R's of radiobiology revisited. Stem Cells. 2010;28(4):639–48. https://doi.org/10.1002/stem.318.
8. Santacroce A, Kamp MA, Budach W, Hänggi D. Radiobiology of radiosurgery for the central nervous system. Biomed Res Int. 2013;2013:362761. https://doi.org/10.1155/2013/362761. Epub 2013 Dec 29
9. Brown PD, Ahluwalia MS, Khan OH, Asher AL, Wefel JS, Gondi V. Whole-brain radiotherapy for brain metastases: evolution or revolution? J Clin Oncol. 2018;36(5):483–91. https://doi.org/10.1200/JCO.2017.75.9589.
10. Mizumoto M, Oshiro Y, Yamamoto T, Kohzuki H, Sakurai H. Proton beam therapy for pediatric brain tumor. Neurol Med Chir (Tokyo). 2017;57(7):343–55. https://doi.org/10.2176/nmc.ra.2017-0003.
11. Ruggi A, Melchionda F, Sardi I, Pavone R, Meneghello L, Kitanovski L, Zaletel LZ, Farace P, Zucchelli M, Scagnet M, Toni F, Righetto R, Cianchetti M, Prete A, Greto D, Cammelli S, Morganti AG, Rombi B. Toxicity and clinical results after proton therapy for pediatric Medulloblastoma: a multi-centric retrospective study. Cancers (Basel). 2022;14(11):2747. https://doi.org/10.3390/cancers14112747.

Chapter 10
Immunotherapy

Joe M Das

1. Which of the following cells is involved in critical functions including cytotoxicity, phagocytosis, and T-cell activation through antigen presentation?

    (a) Oligodendroglia
    (b) Microglia
    (c) Astrocyte
    (d) NG2-glia

    Answer: b

2. Which of the following is false regarding NG2-glia?

    (a) Expresses surface chondroitin sulfate proteoglycan 3
    (b) First described as progenitors for oligodendrocytes
    (c) They retain their proliferative ability throughout life
    (d) They help to repair the brain in demyelinating diseases

    Answer: a

    NG2 cells = oligodendrocyte precursor cells (OPCs) = polydendrocytes.

    Key features of neuron-glia antigen 2 (NG2) glia:

    • Expression of surface chondroitin sulfate proteoglycan 4
    • First described as progenitors for oligodendrocytes
    • Recognized as a fourth neuroglial cell type in the mammalian central nervous system
    • Retain their proliferative ability throughout life
    • Maintenance of neuronal function and survival by regulating the neuroimmunological functions in the mature CNS

J. M. Das (✉)
Consultant Neurosurgeon, Bahrain Specialist Hospital, Juffair, Bahrain
e-mail: neurosurgeon@doctors.org.uk

J. M. Das, *Neuro-Oncology Explained Through Multiple Choice Questions*,
https://doi.org/10.1007/978-3-031-13253-7_10

- NG2 glia helps in brain repair in demyelinating disease by proliferating and differentiating into myelinating oligodendrocytes.

3. What is the purpose of the immune reaction in CNS pathology?

   (a) To activate microglia
   (b) To promote phagocytosis
   (c) To stimulate the production of oligodendrocytes
   (d) To allow neurons to function undisturbed

   Answer: d

4. Which of the following is the most selective barrier for limiting the entry of different substances into the brain?

   (a) Blood-meningeal barrier
   (b) Blood-brain barrier
   (c) Choroid plexus barrier
   (d) Blood-CSF barrier

   Answer: b

   - Blood-brain barrier (BBB)—Between the vasculature of the brain parenchyma and the brain parenchyma itself
   - Blood-meningeal barrier (BMB)- Barrier between the meningeal blood vessels and the meninges themselves
   - Choroid plexus barrier (blood-CSF barrier—BCSFB)—Prevents the entry of molecules in the blood into the ventricular CSF.
   - Immune cells can cross the BCSFB and the BMB as the endothelial cells are fenestrated.

5. The primary site of entry of immune cells in pathological states is via

   (a) Blood-meningeal barrier
   (b) Blood-brain barrier
   (c) Choroid plexus barrier
   (d) Blood-CSF barrier

   Answer: a

   - Immune cells will enter primarily via the meningeal vessels across the BMB into the pia and infiltrates the cerebral parenchyma when there is a pathological condition.

6. Which of the following is false regarding dendritic cells in relation to the central nervous system?

   (a) They are typically not found in normal brain parenchyma
   (b) They are present in the choroid plexus and meninges
   (c) They do not secrete IFN alfa
   (d) They migrate to the brain and spinal cord via afferent lymphatics or high endothelial venules

   Answer: c

- Normal dendritic cells secrete IFNα that helps in T-cell maturation, whereas brain tumor-associated dendritic cells will not secrete IFNα.

7. Which of the following does not usually correlate with an improved prognosis is glioblastoma?

   (a) Increased calreticulin
   (b) Increased HSP70
   (c) Decreased HMGB1
   (d) Decreased ratio of infiltrated CD8+ to CD4+ T-cells

   Answer: d

   Damage-Associated Molecular Patterns (DAMPs):

- Increased calreticulin
- Increased HSP70
- Decreased HMGB1

8. Match the following vaccines with the corresponding types

(a) Peptide vaccine	Ofranergene obadenovec (ofra-vec; VB-111)
(b) Dendritic cell vaccine	Ipilimumab (anti–CTLA-4 mAb)
(c) Immune checkpoint inhibitor	Rindopepimut®
(d) Non-replicative viral therapy	Sipuleucel-T

   Answer:

(a) Peptide vaccine	Rindopepimut®
(b) Dendritic cell vaccine	Sipuleucel-T
(c) Immune checkpoint inhibitor	Ipilimumab (anti–CTLA-4 mAb)
(d) Non-replicative viral therapy	Ofranergene obadenovec (ofra-vec; VB-111)

- Ipilimumab—a monoclonal antibody inhibitor for cytotoxic T-lymphocyte–associated protein type 4 (CTLA-4) used to treat stage IV melanoma
- Sipuleucel-T (Provenge®)—dendritic cell vaccine—used to treat stage IV metastatic castrate-resistant prostate cancer.

9. What is the molecular target for Rindopepimut®?

   (a) EGFRvIII
   (b) FGFR
   (c) Hepatocyte Growth Factor Receptor (MET)
   (d) Sprouty2 (SPRY2)

   Answer: a

- Rindopepimut® (CDX-110) is a peptide vaccine used for brain tumors. Trials have shown a mixed response to this drug.
- Peptide vaccine → In vivo dendritic cell maturation → Promotes the production of activated T-cells → Antigen presentation to T-cells → Brain cancer cell damage

10. The most common target for antibody-based drugs for GBM is

   (a) VEGF-A
   (b) Programmed cell death protein 1 (PD-1)
   (c) Cytotoxic T-lymphocyte-associated antigen 4 (CTLA-4)
   (d) HER-2

   Answer: a

11. Which of the following is a Programmed cell death—ligand 1 (PD-L1) inhibitor that is being studied for the treatment of glioblastoma?

   (a) Nivolumab
   (b) Cemiplimab
   (c) Pembrolizumab
   (d) Atezolizumab

   Answer: d

   • Nivolumab, cemiplimab, and pembrolizumab—Anti–PD-1 (programmed death—1) monoclonal antibodies
   • Atezolizumab, durvalumab, and avelumab—PD-L1 inhibitors

12. The recombinant oncolytic poliovirus, PVS-RIPO, is administered through which route?

   (a) Intraventricular
   (b) Intratumoral
   (c) Intravenous
   (d) Intraarterial

   Answer: b

   • PVS-RIPO contains recombinant, live-attenuated type 1 (Sabin) poliovirus vaccine.
   • Carries internal ribosomal entry site (IRES) of human rhinovirus 2.
   • Enters the neoplastic cells via the polio receptor CD155, expressed in solid tumors.
   • Has found initial promise in patients with recurrent glioblastoma.

13. Neurons support tumor cell proliferation via secretion of

   (a) Neuroligin-1
   (b) Neuroligin-2
   (c) Neuroligin-3
   (d) Neuroligin-4

   Answer: c

   • NLGN3 expression strongly predicts survival in human high-grade gliomas.

14. Indolamine 2,3-dioxygenase 1 (IDO) which is known to suppress the anti-glioblastoma immune response is involved in the metabolism of which of the following amino acids?

(a) Glycine
(b) Glutamine
(c) Tyrosine
(d) Tryptophan

Answer: d

- Tryptophan is the least abundant amino acid.
- IDO1 converts tryptophan into kynure nines.
- Navoximod and linrodostat are IDO inhibitors being tried in preclinical models of glioblastoma.
- Indoximod, another IDO inhibitor, is being tried in pediatric brain tumors.

15. Which of the following DNA viruses has shown promising results in the treatment of gliomas?

(a) Reovirus
(b) Newcastle Disease Virus (NDV)
(c) Measles virus
(d) Adenovirus

Answer: d

- The following viruses have shown promising results in oncolytic therapy of gliomas:
  - DNA viruses: Modified HSV1, Adenovirus
  - RNA viruses: Reovirus, NDV

16. The most abundant cell types in the tumor mass of glioblastoma are

(a) Astrocytes
(b) Tumor-associated macrophages
(c) Neutrophils
(d) Oligodendrocytes

Answer: b

- Tumor-associated macrophages (TAMs) are the most abundant cells in the GBM microenvironment,
- CD11b, also known as integrin alpha M, is often used to identify TAMs.
- CD14 is widely used for human TAMs.

17. The glymphatic system is a brain-wide perivascular pathway driven by which of the following aquaporins?

(a) Aquaporin 1
(b) Aquaporin 2

    (c) Aquaporin 3
    (d) Aquaporin 4

    Answer: d

    "Glymphatic system" was discovered in 2012 by Iliff et al.
    It helps in:

- Clearing the interstitial solutes in the brain parenchyma
- Para-arterial influx of subarachnoisd CSF into the brain interstitium,
- Exchanging of CSF with interstitial fluid
- Para-venous efflux of ISF

Test your learning and check your understanding of this book's contents: use the "Springer Nature Flashcards" app to access questions using https://sn.pub/3HwHCw To use the app, please follow the instructions in Chap. 1.

Bibliography

1. Lyon JG, Mokarram N, Saxena T, Carroll SL, Bellamkonda RV. Engineering challenges for brain tumor immunotherapy. Adv Drug Deliv Rev. 2017;114:19–32. https://doi.org/10.1016/j.addr.2017.06.006.
2. Jin X, Riew TR, Kim HL, Choi JH, Lee MY. Morphological characterization of NG2 glia and their association with neuroglial cells in the 3-nitropropionic acid-lesioned striatum of rat. Sci Rep. 2018;8(1):5942–17. https://doi.org/10.1038/s41598-018-24385-0.
3. Srivastava S, Jackson C, Kim T, Choi J, Lim M. A characterization of dendritic cells and their role in immunotherapy in glioblastoma: from preclinical studies to clinical trials. Cancers (Basel). 2019;11(4):537. https://doi.org/10.3390/cancers11040537.
4. Hernandez C, Huebener P, Schwabe RF. Damage-associated molecular patterns in cancer: a double-edged sword. Oncogene. 2016;35(46):5931–41. https://doi.org/10.1038/onc.2016.104.
5. Muth C, Rubner Y, Semrau S, Rühle PF, Frey B, Strnad A, Buslei R, Fietkau R, Gaipl US. Primary glioblastoma multiforme tumors and recurrence: comparative analysis of the danger signals HMGB1, HSP70, and calreticulin. Strahlenther Onkol. 2016;192(3):146–55. https://doi.org/10.1007/s00066-015-0926-z.
6. Han S, Zhang C, Li Q, Dong J, Liu Y, Huang Y, Jiang T, Wu A. Tumour-infiltrating CD4(+) and CD8(+) lymphocytes as predictors of clinical outcome in glioma. Br J Cancer. 2014;110(10):2560–8.
7. Swartz AM, Li QJ, Sampson JH. Rindopepimut: a promising immunotherapeutic for the treatment of glioblastoma multiforme. Immunotherapy. 2014;6(6):679–90. https://doi.org/10.2217/imt.14.21.
8. Razpotnik R, Novak N, Čurin Šerbec V, Rajcevic U. Targeting malignant brain tumors with antibodies. Front Immunol. 2017;8:1181. https://doi.org/10.3389/fimmu.2017.01181.
9. Khasraw M, Reardon DA, Weller M, Sampson JH. PD-1 inhibitors: do they have a future in the treatment of glioblastoma? Clin Cancer Res. 2020;26(20):5287–96. https://doi.org/10.1158/1078-0432.CCR-20-1135. Epub 2020 Jun 11
10. Beasley GM, Nair SK, Farrow NE, Landa K, Selim MA, Wiggs CA, Jung SH, Bigner DD, True Kelly A, Gromeier M, Salama AK. Phase I trial of intratumoral PVSRIPO in patients with unresectable, treatment-refractory melanoma. J Immunother Cancer. 2021;9(4):e002203. https://doi.org/10.1136/jitc-2020-002203.

11. Venkatesh HS, Johung TB, Caretti V, Noll A, Tang Y, Nagaraja S, Gibson EM, Mount CW, Polepalli J, Mitra SS, Woo PJ, Malenka RC, Vogel H, Bredel M, Mallick P, Monje M. Neuronal activity promotes glioma growth through Neuroligin-3 secretion. Cell. 2015;161(4):803–16. https://doi.org/10.1016/j.cell.2015.04.012. Epub 2015 Apr 23

12. Mohan AA, Tomaszewski WH, Haskell-Mendoza AP, Hotchkiss KM, Singh K, Reedy JL, Fecci PE, Sampson JH, Khasraw M. Targeting immunometabolism in glioblastoma. Front Oncol. 2021;11:696402. https://doi.org/10.3389/fonc.2021.696402.

13. Zhai L, Lauing KL, Chang AL, Dey M, Qian J, Cheng Y, Lesniak MS, Wainwright DA. The role of IDO in brain tumor immunotherapy. J Neuro-Oncol. 2015;123(3):395–403. https://doi.org/10.1007/s11060-014-1687-8.

14. Rius-Rocabert S, García-Romero N, García A, Ayuso-Sacido A, Nistal-Villan E. Oncolytic Virotherapy in glioma tumors. Int J Mol Sci. 2020;21(20):7604. https://doi.org/10.3390/ijms21207604.

15. Andersen JK, Miletic H, Hossain JA. Tumor-associated macrophages in gliomas-basic insights and treatment opportunities. Cancers (Basel). 2022;14(5):1319. https://doi.org/10.3390/cancers14051319.

16. Xu D, Zhou J, Mei H, Li H, Sun W, Xu H. Impediment of cerebrospinal fluid drainage through Glymphatic system in glioma. Front Oncol. 2022;11:790821. https://doi.org/10.3389/fonc.2021.790821.

Chapter 11
Stem Cells

Joe M Das

1. Which of the following is an example of a suicide gene that is carried by neural stem cells during their administration to prevent their uncontrolled proliferation?

   (a) Fumarase
   (b) Thymidine kinase
   (c) Aconitase
   (d) DNA helicase

   Answer: b

   Usual strategies to induce cell suicide include:

   - Cytosine deaminase gene of *E. coli* (converts 5-Fluorocytosine to 5-Fluorouracil)
   - Herpes simplex virus thymidine kinase gene (converts ganciclovir to ganciclovir monophosphate) → Delay in S phase and G2-phase → Apoptosis

2. Which type of stem cell is closest to the ependymal layer of the ventricle in the subventricular zone?

   (a) Type A
   (b) Type B
   (c) Type C
   (d) Type D

   Answer: a

J. M. Das (✉)
Consultant Neurosurgeon, Bahrain Specialist Hospital, Juffair, Bahrain
e-mail: neurosurgeon@doctors.org.uk

© The Author(s), under exclusive license to Springer Nature Switzerland AG 2023
J. M. Das, *Neuro-Oncology Explained Through Multiple Choice Questions*,
https://doi.org/10.1007/978-3-031-13253-7_11

- Adult neural stem cells (NSCs) are present in:

  - The subventricular zone (SVZ) of the lateral ventricles and
  - The subgranular layer of the hippocampal dentate gyrus.

- NSCs (quiescent type B cells) → rapidly dividing type C cells → type A cells (neuroblasts)
- Type A cells are separated only by a single layer of ependymal cells.
- Type A cells directly divide to form new neurons.

3. The most likely location of glioma stem cell (GSC) niche in which the GSC reside is around which of the following type of blood vessels?

   (a) Arteriole
   (b) Venule
   (c) Capillary
   (d) Venous sinus

   Answer: a

   GSC niches

   - The protective microenvironments in glioblastomas
   - Hypoxic
   - Located in a periarteriolar fashion

4. Which is the most developed brain tumor stem cell marker?

   (a) Prominin-1
   (b) Sox2
   (c) Nestin
   (d) Musashi1

   Answer: a

   Prominin-1 (Cluster of Differentiation 133—CD133):

   - Pentaspan transmembrane glycoprotein
   - Located on cell protrusions
   - Detected in patients with familial macular degeneration
   - First used to enrich tumor-populating cells in leukemia
       Nestin and CD133: the most sensitive markers for both adult NSCs and BTSCs.

5. Which of the following is the best-known RNA marker that is associated with the progression of glioblastoma?

   (a) ψ
   (b) m^1A
   (c) m^6A
   (d) m^6A_m

   Answer: c

- RNA modifications = RNA epigenetics
- Present in almost all the cellular RNAs.
- N6-methyladenosine (m^6A) modification: essential for tumor development
- Most prevalent and abundant modification that occurs in mRNAs, rRNAs, and snRNAs.
- Occurs in nuclear speckles

RNA markers elevated in glioblastoma:

- m6A writers: WTAP and RBM15
- m6A eraser: ALKBH5
- m6A reader: YTHDF2

RNA markers decreased in glioblastoma:

- m6A writers: METTL3, VIRMA, and ZC3H13
- m6A eraser: FTO
- m6A readers: YTHDC2 and hnRNPC

6. Which of the following drugs inhibits the SHH-GLI pathway and reduces the growth of human medulloblastomas and gliomas?

    (a) Cyclopamine
    (b) BMP
    (c) Bevacizumab
    (d) STAT3

   Answer: a

   SHH inhibitor—Inhibits stem cell proliferation.
   Differentiation therapy—BMP—Depletes stem cells.
   Anti-angiogenic therapy—Bevacizumab—Disrupts angiogenic niche.
   STAT3

- Pro-survival and pro-inflammatory transcription factor
- Abnormally active in GBM
- A master regulator of tumorigenesis
- A mediator of therapeutic resistance

7. Which of the following cyclins is the chief promoter of the proliferation of stem cells in the subventricular zone?

    (a) Cyclin D1
    (b) Cyclin D2
    (c) Cyclin D3
    (d) Cyclin D4

   Answer: b

- Three D-type cyclins—Cyclin D1, D2, and D3
- Checkpoint regulators of the human cell cycle

- Promote the transition from G1 to S phase through:

  – Activation of the cyclin-dependent kinase Cdk4/6
  – Phosphorylation of retinoblastoma suppressor protein (pRB)
  – Suppression of pRB inhibitory function on E2F transcription factors

- Cyclin D2—predominant cyclin D in the human subventricular zone

8. Which of the following glioma stem cell markers is expressed in Down syndrome?

   (a) CD44
   (b) SOX2
   (c) Nestin
   (d) Olig2

   Answer: d

   Stem cell markers expressed in glioblastoma—CD44, SOX2, Nestin, and Olig2.

- **CD44**

  – Surface glycoprotein—chromosome 11
  – A marker for CNS development and malignant transformation to gliomas
  – Also prognostic

- **SOX2**

  – Transcription factor—chromosome 3
  – Maintains the self-renewal capacity of undifferentiated stem cells

- **Nestin**

  – Type IV intermediate filament—NE gene (19q23.1)
  – Responsible for the mechanical integrity of the cell
  – Expressed in nerve cells during the initial phase of development

- **OLIG2**

  – Transcription factor—gene 21q22.11
  – Defines oligodendroglial differentiation
  – Anti-neurogenic or pro-neurogenic during different stages of CNS development
  – Expressed in Down syndrome and CNS tumors (Glioblastomas, astrocytomas, and oligodendrogliomas)

9. Which of the following is not a definitive functional characteristic of a cancer stem cell?

   (a) Sustained self-renewal
   (b) Persistent proliferation

(c) Tumor initiation upon secondary transplantation

(d) Stem cell marker expression

Answer: d

Cancer stem cells share some common features with somatic stem cells.

- Frequency within the tumor
- Ability to generate progeny of multiple lineages
- Stem cell marker expression

10. Which of the following stem cell type is characterized by the generation of a tumor, which lacks the capacity for self-renewal, upon secondary transplantation?

(a) Cancer stem cell

(b) Cancer stem-like cell

(c) Cancer-initiating cell

(d) Cancer-propagating cell

Answer: c

11. Which is a cytoplasmic protein delineated as a cancer stem cell marker?

(a) Musashi-1

(b) Oc4

(c) Nanog

(d) Sox2

Answer: a

Cancer Stem Cells:

- Glycans attached to cell surface proteins or lipids:

  – CD133, CD44, CD15, CD24, CD90, CD49f, CXCR4, L1CAM and ABC efflux transporters.

- Cytoplasmic proteins:

  – Nestin, Musashi-1, and aldehyde dehydrogenase (ALDH1)

- Nuclear proteins:

  – Oc 4, Nanog, and Sox2

12. What is the cut-off of molecular weight and the number of hydrogen bonds In a molecule to be able to cross the blood-brain barrier by lipid-mediated diffusion?

(a) Molecular weight < 100 Da and < 2 hydrogen bonds

(b) Molecular weight < 200 Da and < 4 hydrogen bonds

(c) Molecular weight < 300 Da and < 6 hydrogen bonds

(d) Molecular weight < 400 Da and < 8 hydrogen bonds

Answer: d

13. Match the following molecules with the corresponding mechanisms of action.

(a) Cyclopamine	STAT3 inhibitor
(b) Resveratrol	Induces stem cell differentiation
(c) Metformin	Shh inhibition
(d) Napabucasin	Permeability glycoprotein inhibitor
(e) Epigallocatechin gallate	Activates autophagy
(f) Curcumin	Modulates the Wnt pathway
(g) Bone Morphogenetic Protein 4 (BMP4)	Inhibits AKT signaling

Answer:

(a) Cyclopamine	Shh inhibition
(b) Resveratrol	Modulates the Wnt pathway
(c) Metformin	Inhibits AKT signaling
(d) Napabucasin	STAT3 inhibitor
(e) Epigallocatechin gallate	Permeability glycoprotein inhibitor
(f) Curcumin	Activates autophagy
(g) Bone Morphogenetic Protein 4 (BMP4)	Induces stem cell differentiation

14. Which is a highly selective aurora-A kinase inhibitor that inhibits colony formation in glioma stem cells and potentiates the effects of temozolomide and radiation in glioblastoma?

(a) Honokiol
(b) Alisertib
(c) Pazopanib
(d) Cyclopamine

Answer: b

- Honokiol—Inhibits PI3K/mTOR signaling activation in gliomas
- Pazopanib—Oral multitarget angiogenesis inhibitor
- Cyclopamine—Specifically inhibits the Hedgehog pathway

15. As of now, which of the following neural stem cell lines has been approved for human clinical trials in glioblastoma?

(a) HB1.F3.CD
(b) ReNCell VM
(c) ReNCell CX
(d) Hoechst 33342 SP

Answer: a

Test your learning and check your understanding of this book's contents: use the "Springer Nature Flashcards" app to access questions using https://sn.pub/3HwHCw To use the app, please follow the instructions in Chap. 1.

Bibliography

1. Bexell D, Svensson A, Bengzon J. Stem cell-based therapy for malignant glioma. Cancer Treat Rev. 2013;39(4):358–65. https://doi.org/10.1016/j.ctrv.2012.06.006.
2. Zarogoulidis P, Darwiche K, Sakkas A, Yarmus L, Huang H, Li Q, Freitag L, Zarogoulidis K, Malecki M. Suicide gene therapy for cancer - current strategies. J Genet Syndr Gene Ther. 2013;9(4):16849. https://doi.org/10.4172/2157-7412.1000139.
3. Dong Z, Cui H. The emerging roles of RNA modifications in glioblastoma. Cancers (Basel). 2020;12(3):736. https://doi.org/10.3390/cancers12030736.
4. Alves ALV, Gomes INF, Carloni AC, Rosa MN, da Silva LS, Evangelista AF, Reis RM, Silva VAO. Role of glioblastoma stem cells in cancer therapeutic resistance: a perspective on antineoplastic agents from natural sources and chemical derivatives. Stem Cell Res Ther. 2021;12(1):206. https://doi.org/10.1186/s13287-021-02231-x.
5. Calinescu AA, Kauss MC, Sultan Z, Al-Holou WN, O'Shea SK. Stem cells for the treatment of glioblastoma: a 20-year perspective. CNS. Oncologia. 2021;10(2):CNS73. https://doi.org/10.2217/cns-2020-0026.
6. Rich JN, Eyler CE. Cancer stem cells in brain tumor biology. Cold Spring Harb Symp Quant Biol. 2008;73:411–20. https://doi.org/10.1101/sqb.2008.73.060. Epub 2009 Mar 27

Chapter 12
Nanotheranostics

Joe M Das

1. What is meant by theranostic nanomedicine?

    (a) Nanomedicine combined with diagnostics
    (b) Nanomedicine combined with therapeutics
    (c) Nanomedicine combined with diagnostics and therapeutics
    (d) Nanomedicine combined with teratology

    Answer: c

   - Nanotheranostics:

      – Injection of the nanotheranostic agent *via* different drug particles → reaches the target area of the body → the shell of the medicine disintegrates → release of the agent

   - Nanocapsules—vesicular systems in which a drug is confined to a cavity surrounded by a polymer membrane
   - Nanospheres—matrix systems in which the drug is physically and uniformly dispersed.

2. The only theranostic tool approved for use in the clinical treatment of glioblastoma in Europe consists of nanoparticles, the cores of which are formed by

    (a) Fe_3O_2
    (b) Fe_2O_3
    (c) Fe_3O_4
    (d) Fe_4O_3

    Answer: c

J. M. Das (✉)
Consultant Neurosurgeon, Bahrain Specialist Hospital, Juffair, Bahrain
e-mail: neurosurgeon@doctors.org.uk

© The Author(s), under exclusive license to Springer Nature
Switzerland AG 2023
J. M. Das, *Neuro-Oncology Explained Through Multiple Choice Questions*,
https://doi.org/10.1007/978-3-031-13253-7_12

- The only theranostic tool approved for use in the clinical treatment of glioblastoma in Europe is the magnetic fluid MFL AS-1 (NanoTherm®, MagForce AG, Berlin, Germany).
- Aqueous dispersion of superparamagnetic nanoparticles.
- An iron concentration of 112 mg/ml.
- Nanoparticles are formed as magnetite (Fe_3O_4) cores of approx. 12 nm diameter
- Coating is given by aminosilane, an inert, enzymatically not cleavable silicium compound with a positively charged surface.
- This product is applied directly on the tumor either stereotactically or post-resection.
- Externally applied alternating magnetic field creates heat through relaxation processes.

3. Which of the following is the most used quantum dot nanomaterial for diagnostic purposes?

(a) Polydentate phosphine-coated QDs
(b) Cadmium selenide/Zinc sulfide (CdSe@ZnS)
(c) Nitrogen and sulfur co-doped carbon dots (N,S/CDs)
(d) Polyacrylic acid-coated $Cu_2(OH)PO_4$ quantum dots ($Cu_2(OH) PO_4$@PAA QDs)

Answer: b

4. Which of the following nanoparticles has a low chance of producing cytotoxicity?

(a) Gold nanoparticles
(b) Magnetic nanoparticles
(c) Quantum dots
(d) Carbon nanotubes

Answer: a

- Gold nanoparticles—Low cytotoxicity—2–60 nm
- Magnetic nanoparticles—Potential cytotoxicity—7–20 nm
- Quantum dots—Potential cytotoxicity—2–50 nm
- Carbon nanotubes—Potential cytotoxicity—0.4–40 nm

5. **Match the following lipid-based nanosystems with their composition**

(a) Niosomes	Solid lipid, emulsifier, and water/solvent.
(b) Cubosomes	Nanostructured liquid crystalline particles
(c) Cubosomes and hexosomes	Physiological and biocompatible lipids, surfactants, and co-surfactants.
(d) Transferosomes	Biodegradable natural or synthetic phospholipids.
(e) Ethosomes	Unsaturated long-chain monoglycerides emulsified in water

(f) Liposomes	Nonionic surfactants
(g) Monoolein aqueous dispersion	Phospholipids, alcohol, and water
(h) Solid lipid nanoparticles (SLNs)	Phosphatidylcholine and an edge activator
(i) Nanostructured lipid carriers (NLCs)	Lipid cubic phase and stabilized by a polymer-based outer corona.

Answer:

(a) Niosomes	Nonionic surfactants
(b) Cubosomes	Lipid cubic phase and stabilized by a polymer-based outer corona.
(c) Cubosomes and hexosomes	Nanostructured liquid crystalline particles
(d) Transferosomes	Phosphatidylcholine and an edge activator
(e) Ethosomes	Phospholipids, alcohol, and water.
(f) Liposomes	Biodegradable natural or synthetic phospholipids
(g) Monoolein aqueous dispersion	Unsaturated long-chain monoglycerides emulsified in water
(h) Solid lipid nanoparticles (SLNs)	Solid lipid, emulsifier, and water/solvent
(i) Nanostructured lipid carriers (NLCs)	Physiological and biocompatible lipids, surfactants, and co-surfactants.

6. Which of the following are nano-sized, radially symmetric molecules with a well-defined, homogeneous, and monodisperse structures consisting of tree-like arms or branches?

(a) Carbon nanotubes
(b) Dendrimers
(c) Quantum dots
(d) Metal organic frameworks

Answer: b

Quantum Dots (QDs)

- Nanoscale semiconductor crystals
- First described by Ekimov and Onushenko
- Ranging between 1 and 10 nm in size
- Possess optical and electronic properties different from those of larger particles of bulk material, due to quantum mechanics.

Metal Organic Frameworks (MOFs)

- Crystalline porous solids
- Composed of a three-dimensional (3D) network of metal ions
- Held in place by multidentate organic molecules

Carbon Nanotubes (CNTs)

- Cylinder-shaped allotropic forms of carbon
- Most widely produced under chemical vapor deposition

7. Which is the most widely used magnetic nanoparticle that has intrinsic imaging properties for T_2 contrast?

   (a) Gold
   (b) Iron oxide
   (c) Manganese oxide
   (d) Gadolinium

   Answer: b

   • Manganese and Gadolinium are T1-contrast agents.

8. Which of the following medicines helps to induce radiosensitivity in glioma stem cells (bearing CD133) by inhibiting the Notch signaling pathway?

   (a) α-secretase inhibitor
   (b) β-secretase inhibitor
   (c) γ-secretase inhibitor
   (d) δ-secretase inhibitor

   Answer: c

9. What is a nanoparticle?

   (a) A particle with at least one dimension smaller than 100 nanometers (nm)
   (b) A particle with at least two dimensions smaller than 100 nm
   (c) A particle with all three dimensions smaller than 100 nm
   (d) A particle with all three dimensions smaller than 1 nm

   Answer: a

   Nanoparticles are classified into:

   • Inorganic—Metallic, non-metallic
   • Organic—Organic lipid nanomaterials, organic polymeric nanomaterials

10. What is the optimum size for nanoparticles to avoid immediate clearance by the lymphatic system?

    (a) 100 nm
    (b) 200 nm
    (c) 300 nm
    (d) 400 nm

    Answer: a

    Nanoparticle with a size of 100 nm→

    • Restricted nanoparticle accumulation around tumor blood vessels
    • Poor penetration into the tumor parenchyma

    Nanoparticles <10 nm are cleared by renal excretion and phagocytosis.

11. Optoacoustic imaging, also known as photoacoustic imaging, is based on what principle?

   (a) Light-in, sound-in
   (b) Light-out, sound-out
   (c) Light-in, sound-out
   (d) Light-out, sound-in

    Answer: c

- Nanoparticles can be loaded with small-molecule organic dyes with high photothermic conversion efficiency, eg. IR780 or ICG, to make them imageable.

12. NBTXR3, used in Computed Tomography nanotheranostics is composed of

   (a) Magnesium oxide
   (b) Manganese oxide
   (c) Hafnium oxide
   (d) Zirconium oxide

    Answer: c

    NBTXR3

- Hafnium oxide (HfO_2) crystalline nanoparticles
- Functionalized with anionic phosphate coating
- 50 nm size
- Acts as radioenhancers to increase energy deposition in the tumor during radiotherapy
- CT contrasts allows visualization of their accumulation in tumors.

13. Which is the most promising protein for the synthesis of carbon quantum dots?

   (a) Albumin
   (b) Globulin
   (c) Myosin
   (d) Keratin

    Answer: a

    Carbon Quantum Dots

- Special class of carbon nanomaterial
- Made up of carbon nanoparticles
- Size <10 nm

14. What is the size of an ultra small superparamagnetic iron oxide nanoparticle (USPION)?

   (a) <10 nm
   (b) 10–50 nm

(c) 50–180 nm
(d) >180 nm

Answer: b

- Superparamagnetic iron oxide nanoparticle (SPION)—50–180 nm
- Ultra small superparamagnetic iron oxide nanoparticle (USPION)—10–50 nm
- Very small superparamagnetic iron oxide nanoparticle (SPION)—<10 nm

15. Which compound is tried as a radiosensitizer and MRI contrast-enhancing nanoparticle?

(a) AGuIX
(b) Manganese oxide
(c) Lipid-coated perfluoropropane
(d) Magnesium oxide

Answer: a

AGuIX (Activation and Guidance of Irradiation by X-ray)

- Sub-5 nm nanoparticles
- Composed of a polysiloxane matrix with gadolinium cyclic chelates
- Covalently grafted on inorganic matrix

The commercial organic microbubbles or liposomes used in ultrasound imaging are lipid-coated perfluoropropane microbubbles—Phase transition temperature of 56 °C.

Test your learning and check your understanding of this book's contents: use the "Springer Nature Flashcards" app to access questions using https://sn.pub/3HwHCw To use the app, please follow the instructions in Chap. 1.

Bibliography

1. Zhang P, Zhang L, Qin Z, Hua S, Guo Z, Chu C, et al. Genetically engineered liposome-like nanovesicles as active targeted transport platform. Adv Mater. 2018;30:1705350. https://doi.org/10.1002/adma.201705350.
2. Muthu MS, Leong DT, Mei L, Feng SS. Nanotheranostics - application and further development of nanomedicine strategies for advanced theranostics. Theranostics. 2014;4(6):660–77. https://doi.org/10.7150/thno.8698.
3. Martinelli C, Pucci C, Ciofani G. Nanostructured carriers as innovative tools for cancer diagnosis and therapy. APL Bioeng. 2019;3(1):011502. https://doi.org/10.1063/1.5079943.
4. d'Angelo M, Castelli V, Benedetti E, et al. Theranostic nanomedicine for malignant gliomas. Front Bioeng Biotechnol. 2019;7:325. [published correction appears Front Bioeng Biotechnol. 2020 7:468], Published 2019 Nov 14. https://doi.org/10.3389/fbioe.2019.00325.
5. Bozzato E, Bastiancich C, Préat V. Nanomedicine: a useful tool against Glioma stem cells. Cancers (Basel). 2020;13(1):9. https://doi.org/10.3390/cancers13010009.

6. Buzea C, Pacheco II, Robbie K. Nanomaterials and nanoparticles: sources and toxicity. Biointerphases. 2007;2(4):M17–71. https://doi.org/10.1116/1.2815690.
7. Pijeira MSO, Viltres H, Kozempel J, Sakmár M, Vlk M, İlem-Özdemir D, Ekinci M, Srinivasan S, Rajabzadeh AR, Ricci-Junior E, Alencar LMR, Al Qahtani M, Santos-Oliveira R. Radiolabeled nanomaterials for biomedical applications: radiopharmacy in the era of nanotechnology. EJNMMI Radiopharm Chem. 2022;7(1):8. https://doi.org/10.1186/s41181-022-00161-4.
8. Rizvi SA, Saleh AM. Applications of nanoparticle systems in drug delivery technology. Saudi Pharm J. 2018;26(1):64–70. https://doi.org/10.1016/j.jsps.2017.10.012.
9. Zein R, Sharrouf W, Selting K. Physical properties of nanoparticles that result in improved cancer targeting. J Oncol. 2020;2020:1–16. https://doi.org/10.1155/2020/5194780.
10. Barua S, Mitragotri S. Challenges associated with penetration of nanoparticles across cell and tissue barriers: a review of current status and future prospects. Nano Today. 2014;9(2):223–43. https://doi.org/10.1016/j.nantod.2014.04.008.
11. Dennahy IS, Han Z, MacCuaig WM, Chalfant HM, Condacse A, Hagood JM, Claros-Sorto JC, Razaq W, Holter-Chakrabarty J, Squires R, Edil BH, Jain A, McNally LR. Nanotheranostics for image-guided cancer treatment. Pharmaceutics. 2022;14(5):917. https://doi.org/10.3390/pharmaceutics14050917.
12. Naik K, Chaudhary S, Ye L, Parmar AS. A strategic review on carbon quantum dots for cancer-diagnostics and treatment. Front Bioeng Biotechnol. 2022;18(10):882100. https://doi.org/10.3389/fbioe.2022.882100.
13. Cortajarena AL, Ortega D, Ocampo SM, Gonzalez-García A, Couleaud P, Miranda R, Belda-Iniesta C, Ayuso-Sacido A. Engineering iron oxide nanoparticles for clinical settings. Nanobiomedicine (Rij). 2014;1(1):2. https://doi.org/10.5772/58841.

Chapter 13
Metastatic Brain Tumors

Joe M Das

1. The most common underlying cause of brain metastasis is

   (a) Breast cancer
   (b) Prostate cancer
   (c) Lung cancer
   (d) Colorectal cancer

   Answer: c

2. Which malignancy has the strongest propensity to metastasize to the brain?

   (a) Breast cancer
   (b) Choriocarcinoma
   (c) Lung cancer
   (d) Melanoma

   Answer: d

   • Choriocarcinoma, although very rare, is the most common gynecologic tumor to metastasize to the CNS.

3. Which of the following types of metastases is radiosensitive?

   (a) Renal cell carcinoma
   (b) Melanoma
   (c) Sarcoma
   (d) Small cell lung cancer

   Answer: d

J. M. Das (✉)
Consultant Neurosurgeon, Bahrain Specialist Hospital, Juffair, Bahrain
e-mail: neurosurgeon@doctors.org.uk

© The Author(s), under exclusive license to Springer Nature
Switzerland AG 2023
J. M. Das, *Neuro-Oncology Explained Through Multiple Choice Questions*,
https://doi.org/10.1007/978-3-031-13253-7_13

4. Which metastasis is most likely to bleed?

   (a) Breast cancer
   (b) Choriocarcinoma
   (c) Lung cancer
   (d) Melanoma

   Answer: d

   Bleed is common in brain metastasis caused by

   - Melanoma
   - Renal cell carcinoma
   - Choriocarcinoma

5. The most common presentation of brain metastasis is

   (a) Headache
   (b) Seizure
   (c) Neurological deficit
   (d) Cognitive decline

   Answer: a

6. Which drug, in combination with trastuzumab and capecitabine, was the first one to obtain FDA approval for the treatment of patients with breast cancer and brain metastases?

   (a) Acalabrutinib
   (b) Ripretinib
   (c) Pemigatinib
   (d) Tucatinib

   Answer: d

7. Which statement regarding intracranial metastases is false?

   (a) Metastases of small cell lung carcinoma are equally distributed in all regions of the brain
   (b) Pelvic and gastrointestinal tumors commonly metastasize to the posterior fossa
   (c) HER-2–expressing breast cancer also has a higher incidence of brain metastasis compared with HER-2–negative breast cancer.
   (d) Non-small-cell lung cancer is more likely to metastasize to the brain than small-cell lung cancer

   Answer: d

8. Which is not an indication for surgery in brain metastasis?

   (a) Large lesions (>3 cm)
   (b) Fewer than three resectable lesions

   (c) KPS <70

   (d) Limited systemic disease

Answer: c

- KPS > 70 is needed.

9. Supramarginal resection implies the removal of how much of normal-appearing perifocal tissue?

   (a) 1 mm

   (b) 2 mm

   (c) 3 mm

   (d) 5 mm

Answer: c

10. Which is not an FDA-approved indication for Bevacizumab?

   (a) Recurrent glioblastoma

   (b) Advanced non–small cell lung cancer (NSCLC)

   (c) Metastatic renal cell cancer

   (d) Initial diagnosis of glioblastoma

Answer: d

11. The most common form of bleeding linked to bevacizumab is

   (a) Epistaxis

   (b) Hemoptysis

   (c) Intracranial hemorrhage

   (d) Melena

Answer: a

12. What is the treatment of choice for patients with an ECOG performance status of 0–2 and up to 4 intact brain metastases, the largest being <2 cm in size?

   (a) Single fraction SRS

   (b) Multi-fraction SRS

   (c) Surgical resection

   (d) Whole brain radiation therapy

Answer: a

- Single fraction SRS dose—2000–2400 cGy

13. For brain metastases patients having a favorable prognosis and those receiving WBRT or hippocampal avoidance WBRT, the addition of which of the following drugs is recommended?

   (a) Memantine

   (b) Temozolomide

    (c) Bevacizumab

    (d) Dexamethasone

    Answer: a

14. Hippocampal avoidance while administering whole brain radiation therapy is not appropriate in which of the following conditions?

    (a) Patients with favorable prognosis

    (b) Leptomeningeal disease

    (c) Patients with a seizure disorder

    (d) Breast cancer metastases

    Answer: b

- Lesions located close to the hippocampus are another contraindication for hippocampal avoidance.

15. What is the treatment recommendation for a patient with a limited number of brain metastases having an ECOG performance status of 3–4 with stable systemic disease and the largest metastasis measuring <4 cm with no mass effect?

    (a) Single fraction SRS

    (b) Multi-fraction SRS

    (c) Surgical resection

    (d) Whole brain radiation therapy

    Answer: d

- For a patient with a limited number of brain metastases having an ECOG performance status 0–2 with the largest metastasis measuring <2 cm can be managed with single fraction SRS.
- Lesions >4 cm or mass effect need neurosurgical consultation.

WHO Classification of Metastases to the CNS

• Metastases to the brain and spinal cord parenchyma
• Metastases to the meninges

Test your learning and check your understanding of this book's contents: use the "Springer Nature Flashcards" app to access questions using https://sn.pub/3HwHCw To use the app, please follow the instructions in Chap. 1.

Bibliography

1. Morgan AJ, Giannoudis A, Palmieri C. The genomic landscape of breast cancer brain metastases: a systematic review. Lancet Oncol. 2021;22(1):e7–e17. https://doi.org/10.1016/S1470-2045(20)30556-8.
2. Jaray H, Wang MD, Lily C. Brain metastases. Ferri's Clinical Advisor. 2022:271–2.

3. Mayer SA, Marshall RS. Chapter 23: Neuroncology. In: On Call Neurology. Elsevier. p. 358–77.
4. Kotecha R, Ahluwalia MS, Siomin V, McDermott MW. Surgery, stereotactic radiosurgery, and systemic therapy in the Management of Operable Brain Metastasis. Neurol Clin. 2022;40(2):421–36. https://doi.org/10.1016/j.ncl.2021.11.002.
5. Ghiaseddin A, Peters KB. Use of bevacizumab in recurrent glioblastoma. CNS Oncol. 2015;4(3):157–69. https://doi.org/10.2217/cns.15.8.
6. Brem S, Desai A, Bagley SJ, Fan Y, Wong ET. Angiogenesis and brain tumors: scientific principles, current therapy, and future. Youmans Winn Neurol Surg. 140:970–970.e33.
7. Gondi V, Bauman G, Bradfield L, Burri SH, Cabrera AR, Cunningham DA, Eaton BR, Hattangadi-Gluth JA, Kim MM, Kotecha R, Kraemer L, Li J, Nagpal S, Rusthoven CG, Suh JH, Tomé WA, Wang TJC, Zimmer AS, Ziu M, Brown PD. Radiation therapy for brain metastases: an ASTRO clinical practice guideline. Pract Radiat Oncol. 2022;12(4):265–82. https://doi.org/10.1016/j.prro.2022.02.003. S1879-8500(22)00054-6, Epub ahead of print

Chapter 14
Low-Grade Gliomas

Joe M Das

1. Which of the following statements about gliomas is false?

   (a) The 10-year overall survival rate for patients having WHO grade 2 astrocytomas is 35%
   (b) Low-Grade Gliomas (LGGs) are primarily most commonly reported in the frontal lobes, followed by temporal lobes
   (c) LGGs originating in the cerebellar region are associated with a worse prognosis than those originating supratentorially
   (d) The most common initial clinical presentation of patients with LGGs is seizures

   Answer: c

   The only agreed-upon surgical standard for adults with suspected or known supratentorial non–optic pathway LGGs is to obtain a tissue diagnosis before active treatment commences.

2. Which anticonvulsant is preferentially used for the control of seizures in patients with intracranial tumors?

   (a) Phenytoin
   (b) Levetiracetam
   (c) Sodium valproate
   (d) Oxcarbazepine

   Answer: b

J. M. Das (✉)
Consultant Neurosurgeon, Bahrain Specialist Hospital, Juffair, Bahrain
e-mail: neurosurgeon@doctors.org.uk

© The Author(s), under exclusive license to Springer Nature
Switzerland AG 2023
J. M. Das, *Neuro-Oncology Explained Through Multiple Choice Questions*,
https://doi.org/10.1007/978-3-031-13253-7_14

3. Which of the following is used as a biomarker for IDH mutation in gliomas during magnetic resonance spectroscopy?

   (a) L-2-hydroxyglutarate
   (b) d-2-hydroxyglutarate
   (c) Alpha-ketoglutarate
   (d) Beta-ketoglutarate

   Answer: b

4. Before anaplastic progression, LGGs have been shown to grow linearly at a mean velocity of diametric expansion of

   (a) 2 mm / year
   (b) 4 mm / year
   (c) 6 mm / year
   (d) 8 mm / year

   Answer: b

   - Velocity of diametric expansion (VDE) has been used as a measure of tumor growth rate.
   - Tumor volume (V) is measured using axial images and manual segmentation.
   - Mean tumor diameter = $(2 \times V)^{1/3}$
   - VDE is calculated from the linear regression of MTD over time.

5. Which of the following features is not suggestive of a low-grade glioma on MRI?

   (a) High axial diffusivity (AD)
   (b) High radial diffusivity (RD)
   (c) High apparent diffusion coefficient (ADC)
   (d) High regional cerebral blood volume

   Answer: d

6. Which of the following is not a common pattern of the secondary structures of Scherer?

   (a) Perineuronal satellitosis
   (b) Perivascular aggregation
   (c) Subpial condensation
   (d) Pial calcification

   Answer: d

   Patterns of infiltrative growth frequently observed in diffuse gliomas = *secondary structures of Scherer*

   - Perineuronal satellitosis
   - Perivascular aggregation
   - Subpial condensation

7. Which of the following mitotic figures is the cut-off for defining anaplasia in an oligodendroglioma?

(a) 4
(b) 6
(c) 8
(d) 10

Answer: b

> 6 mitotic figures per 10 high-power fields as a generally accepted cut-off for designation of anaplasia.

8. Which is the most common mutation present in IDH-mutant diffuse gliomas?

(a) R132H
(b) R321H
(c) R231H
(d) R312H

Answer: a

- The most common mutation present in approximately 90% of IDH-mutant diffuse gliomas—p.R132H

9. Oligodendroglioma, IDH-mutant and 1p/19q co-deleted is characterized by

(a) Presence of IDH1 or IDH 2 mutation with whole-arm codeletion of 1p and 19q
(b) Presence of IDH1 and IDH 2 mutation with whole-arm codeletion of 1p and 19q
(c) Presence of IDH1 or IDH 2 mutation with whole-arm codeletion of 1p or 19q
(d) Presence of IDH1 and IDH 2 mutation with whole-arm codeletion of 1p or 19q

Answer: a

- *Oligodendroglioma, IDH-mutant and 1p/19q co-deleted*—WHO grade 2 tumor
- Genetically defined by:

   - The presence of either an *IDH1* p.R132 or *IDH2* p.R172 missense mutation +
   - Whole-arm co-deletion of chromosomes 1p and 19q

10. Standard chemotherapeutic regimens for low-grade glioma patients do not include

(a) Procarbazine
(b) Lomustine
(c) Vincristine
(d) Carboplatin

Answer: d

- Standard chemotherapy in diffuse low-grade gliomas includes:
  Alkylating chemotherapeutics—temozolomide and PCV (procarbazine, CCNU or lomustine, and vincristine)

11. Which of the following is a key event in the evolution of IDH-mutant diffuse low-grade gliomas?

    (a) Increased production of 2-hydroxyglutarate
    (b) Decreased production of 2-hydroxyglutarate
    (c) Increased concentration of α-ketoglutarate
    (d) Decreased concentration of β-ketoglutarate

    Answer: a

    - ↑2-hydroxyglutarate and ↓α-ketoglutarate appear to be key events in the evolution of IDH-mutant diffuse low-grade gliomas.

12. Which of the following measures the motor cortex and supplementary motor area activity in the brain leading to voluntary muscle movement?

    (a) Bereitschaftspotential
    (b) Readiness potential
    (c) Premotor potential
    (d) All the above

    Answer: d

13. 5-aminolevulinic acid (5-ALA) is converted to which of the following fluorescent metabolites in the malignant brain tumor cells?

    (a) Porphobilinogen
    (b) Protoporphyrin IX
    (c) Phytochromobilin
    (d) Uroporphyrinogen I

    Answer: b

    - 5-ALA is metabolized to protoporphyrin IX (PPIX), a fluorescent metabolite, inside the malignant tumor cells.
    - This is due to decreased levels of ferrochelatase and selective uptake by ABCB6 (ATP-binding cassette transporter).
    - This product emits violet-red fluorescence after excitation with 405 nm wavelength blue light.
    - PPIX plasma levels peak 4 hours after oral administration of 5-ALA (20 mg/kg).

14. The chicken-wire histopathological appearance of oligodendroglioma is given by

    (a) Cell membranes
    (b) Capillaries
    (c) Calcifications
    (d) Chromatin

    Answer: b

15. Which of the following is not protective against the development of a glioma?

    (a) Eczema
    (b) Asthma
    (c) Psoriasis
    (d) Avoiding cell phones

    Answer: d

    • Immunologic illnesses such as allergic rhinitis, asthma, eczema, and psoriasis remain protective against the risk of developing a glioma.
    • Regular cellular phone use is no longer questioned as a risk factor for developing a glioma.
    • The initial step in the management of patients with suspected diffuse low-grade glioma—surgery to provide a specimen for tissue diagnosis ± cytoreduction.

16. Which of the following is not a risk factor for survival of low-grade glioma based on EORTC 22844 and 22845 trials?

    (a) Age older than 40 years
    (b) Astrocytoma histology
    (c) Tumor crossing the midline
    (d) Seizure at presentation

    Answer: d

    Identified Five Risk Factors for Survival

    • Age older than 40 years
    • Astrocytoma histology
    • Tumor maximum diameter ≥ _6 cm
    • Tumor crossing the midline
    • The presence of neurologic impairments at the time of diagnosis

17. Cortical rim of hyperintensity on T1-weighted images and a stalk-like extension to the adjacent ventricle on T2-weighted images are pathognomonic of

    (a) Astroblastoma
    (b) Angiocentric glioma
    (c) Chordoid glioma
    (d) Pleomorphic xanthoastrocytoma

    Answer: a

18. The most frequently mutated gene in pleomorphic xanthoastrocytoma is

    (a) P53
    (b) EGFR
    (c) BRAF
    (d) NF1

    Answer: c

WHO Classification of Gliomas

Adult-type diffuse gliomas
- Astrocytoma, IDH-mutant
- Oligodendroglioma, IDH-mutant, and 1p/19q-codeleted
- Glioblastoma, IDH-wildtype

Pediatric-type diffuse low-grade gliomas
- Diffuse astrocytoma, MYB- or MYBL1-altered
- Angiocentric glioma
- Polymorphous low-grade neuroepithelial tumor of the young
- Diffuse low-grade glioma, MAPK pathway-altered

Pediatric-type diffuse high-grade gliomas
- Diffuse midline glioma, H3 K27-altered
- Diffuse hemispheric glioma, H3 G34-mutant
- Diffuse pediatric-type high-grade glioma, H3-wildtype and IDH-wildtype
- Infant-type hemispheric glioma

Circumscribed astrocytic gliomas
- Pilocytic astrocytoma
- High-grade astrocytoma with piloid features
- Pleomorphic xanthoastrocytoma
- Subependymal giant cell astrocytoma
- Chordoid glioma
- Astroblastoma, MN1-altered

Test your learning and check your understanding of this book's contents: use the "Springer Nature Flashcards" app to access questions using https://sn.pub/3HwHCw To use the app, please follow the instructions in Chap. 1.

Bibliography

1. Sim HW, Nejad R, Zhang W, Nassiri F, Mason W, Aldape KD, Zadeh G, Chen EX. Tissue 2-Hydroxyglutarate as a biomarker for *Isocitrate dehydrogenase* mutations in gliomas. Clin Cancer Res. 2019;25(11):3366–73. https://doi.org/10.1158/1078-0432.CCR-18-3205. Epub 2019 Feb 18
2. Altieri R, Hirono S, Duffau H, Ducati A, Fontanella MM, La Rocca G, Melcarne A, Panciani PP, Spena G, Garbossa D. Natural history of de novo high grade glioma: first description of growth parabola. J Neurosurg Sci. 2020;64(4):399–403. https://doi.org/10.23736/S0390-5616.17.04067-X.
3. Civita P, Valerio O, Naccarato AG, Gumbleton M, Pilkington GJ. *Satellitosis*, a crosstalk between neurons, vascular structures and neoplastic cells in brain Tumours; early manifestation of invasive behaviour. Cancers (Basel). 2020;12:3720. https://doi.org/10.3390/cancers12123720.
4. Shaikh N, Brahmbhatt N, Kruser TJ, Kam KL, Appin CL, Wadhwani N, Chandler J, Kumthekar P, Lukas RV. Pleomorphic xanthoastrocytoma: a brief review. CNS Oncol. 2019;8(3):CNS39. https://doi.org/10.2217/cns-2019-0009. Epub 2019 Sep 19

Chapter 15
High-Grade Gliomas

Joe M Das

1. Tumor treating fields (TTFields) disrupt tumor cells by emitting alternating electric fields at

    (a) 100 kHz
    (b) 200 kHz
    (c) 500 kHz
    (d) 1000 kHz

    Answer: b

2. TTFields act by which of the following mechanisms?

    (a) Causes cellular blebbing
    (b) Dispersal of septin
    (c) Triggers cytoplasmic stress response
    (d) All the above

    Answer: d

3. The most common sites of occurrence of gliosarcoma are in the following order of frequency

    (a) Frontal > parietal > temporal > occipital lobes
    (b) Frontal > temporal > parietal > occipital lobes
    (c) Temporal > parietal > frontal > occipital lobes
    (d) Temporal > frontal > parietal > occipital lobes

    Answer: c

J. M. Das (✉)
Consultant Neurosurgeon, Bahrain Specialist Hospital, Juffair, Bahrain
e-mail: neurosurgeon@doctors.org.uk

4. Which of the following is not a typical feature of a secondary glioblastoma?

   (a) PTEN mutation
   (b) Associated with mutations in TP52 tumor suppressor gene
   (c) Overexpression of platelet-derived growth factor receptor (PDGFR)
   (d) Loss of heterozygosity of chromosome 10q

   Answer: a

   Primary Glioblastomas

   - Age > 50 years
   - EGFR amplification and mutations
   - Loss of heterozygosity of chromosome 10q
   - Deletion of the phosphatase and tensin homolog on chromosome 10
   - Deletion of chromosome p16

   Secondary Glioblastomas

   - Younger patients
   - Transform over a period of several years into glioblastoma.
   - Less common than primary glioblastomas
   - TP53 tumor suppressor gene mutation
   - Overexpression of platelet-derived growth factor receptor (PDGFR)
   - Abnormalities in the p16 and retinoblastoma (Rb) pathways
   - Loss of heterozygosity of chromosome 10q

5. What is the usual range of MIB-1/Ki-67 labeling index for glioblastomas?

   (a) 5–10%
   (b) 10–20%
   (c) 20–30%
   (d) 30–50%

   Answer: b

6. What is the usual dosage of Temozolomide chemotherapy?

   (a) 100–150 mg/m^2, orally, 5 days per week
   (b) 150–200 mg/m^2, orally, 5 days per week
   (c) 200–250 mg/m^2, orally, 5 days per week
   (d) 250–300 mg/m^2, orally, 5 days per week

   Answer: b

7. Which is the most important prognostic factor for high-grade glioma?

   (a) Age
   (b) Karnofsky Performance Scale score
   (c) The extent of resection
   (d) All the above

   Answer: d

The Most Significant Prognostic Factors for HGG:

- Age
- KPS score
- The extent of resection

8. What is the most common symptom of anaplastic oligodendroglioma?

   (a) Headaches
   (b) Vision changes
   (c) Weakness
   (d) Seizures

   Answer: d

9. Gambogic acid, used as an anti-tumor agent, delivered as a microbubble complex acts by inducing vacuolization-associated cell death. This phenomenon is known as

   (a) Apoptosis
   (b) Paraptosis
   (c) Necroptosis
   (d) Pyroptosis

   Answer: b

   Gambogic acid—polyprenylated xanthone derived from the resin of *Garcinia hanburyi*.
   Kills cancer cells by

   - Paraptosis—vacuolization-associated cell death
   - Apoptosis
   - Megamitochondria formation

10. What is the cut-off diameter of a nanoparticle enabling it to cross the blood-brain barrier?

    (a) <0.4 nm
    (b) <4 nm
    (c) <40 nm
    (d) <400 nm

    Answer: c

11. Glucose transporter 1 uses which of the following methods of transport to facilitate transport across the blood-brain barrier?

    (a) Carrier-mediated transport
    (b) Receptor-mediated transcytosis
    (c) Adsorptive-mediated transcytosis
    (d) Cell-mediated transport

    Answer: a

Carrier-Mediated Transport

- Glucose transporter 1 (GLUT1)
- Monocarboxylate transporter 1 (MCT1)
- Large neutral amino acid transporter 1 (LAT1)
- Cationic amino acid transporter type 1 (CAT1)
- Concentrative nucleoside transporter type 2(CNT2)

Receptor-Mediated Transcytosis

- Transferrin (TfR)
- LDL receptor-related protein 1 and 2 (LRP-1, LRP-2)
- Insulin (InsR)
- Leptin
- Epidermal growth factor
- Tumor necrosis factor

Adsorptive-Mediated Transcytosis

- Cationic substance passing through BBB via electrostatic interaction with the plasma membrane

Cell-Mediated Transport

- Leukocytes directly migrate through the cytoplasm of endothelial cells

12. For people with multiple large metastatic brain tumors, whole-brain radiotherapy remains the standard approach. What is the dose of radiation given in this?

   (a) 30 Gy in 20 fractions
   (b) 30 Gy in 10 fractions
   (c) 60 Gy in 20 fractrions
   (d) 60 Gy in 10 fractions

   Answer: b

13. fMRI uses which of the following as contrast agent?

   (a) Ratio of oxyhemoglobin to deoxyhemoglobin
   (b) Ratio of deoxyhemoglobin to oxyhemoglobin
   (c) Oxyhemoglobin
   (d) Deoxyhemoglobin

   Answer: a

14. Which of the following is not a common feature of IDH-mutant glioma?

   (a) Arises in the frontal lobe
   (b) A unilateral pattern of growth
   (c) Sharp tumor margin
   (d) Brilliant contrast enhancement

   Answer: d

15. Which of the following is a specific radiological marker for astrocytic glioma?

   (a) T2/FLAIR matching
   (b) T2/FLAIR mismatch
   (c) T2/T2* matching
   (d) T2/T2* mismatch

   Answer: b

   • T2–FLAIR mismatch sign—T2-weighted hyperintensity often accompanied by relative hypointensity on fluid-attenuated inversion recovery (FLAIR) sequences.
   • Seen in astrocytoma IDH-mutant CNS WHO grades 2 and 3 tumors.

16. What is the most common location of astrocytoma, IDH-mutant?

   (a) Frontal lobe
   (b) Temporal lobe
   (c) Parietal lobe
   (d) Occipital lobe

   Answer: a

17. The absence of which of the following is a defining feature of IDH-mutant astrocytoma WHO grade 3, that differentiates it from grade 4?

   (a) Hypercellularity
   (b) Nuclear atypia
   (c) Significant mitoses
   (d) Microvascular proliferation and necrosis

   Answer: d

   • Astrocytoma, IDH-mutant, CNS WHO grade 2—A single mitosis or a low mitotic count
   • Astrocytoma, IDH-mutant, CNS WHO grade 3—Hypercellular, multinucleated tumor cells, nuclear atypia, and significant mitosis. Absent microvascular proliferation and necrosis.
   • Astrocytoma, IDH-mutant, CNS WHO grade 4—Focal necrosis or CDKN2A/B homozygous deletion
   • Glioblastoma, IDH-wildtype—Large areas of ischemic necrosis or palisading necrosis

18. Which is not a feature of oligodendroglioma, IDH-mutant and 1p/19q codeleted, CNS WHO grade 3 tumor?

   (a) ≥6 mitoses/10 high-power fields (HPFs)
   (b) Microvascular proliferation
   (c) Necrosis
   (d) Low MIB1 labeling index

   Answer: d

19. Cintredekin besudotox (CB), used for convection-enhanced delivery in malignant glioma, contains which interleukin conjugated to truncated *Pseudomonas* exotoxin?

    (a) IL-4
    (b) IL-6
    (c) IL-10
    (d) IL-13

    Answer: d

20. The most commonly used median prescription dose of stereotactic radiosurgery for recurrent glioblastoma is

    (a) 8 Gy
    (b) 12 Gy
    (c) 16 Gy
    (d) 20 Gy

    Answer: c

21. Which of the following drugs, when administered along with stereotactic radiosurgery, has been shown to improve survival, decrease the incidence of radiation necrosis, and allow safe dose escalation of SRS?

    (a) Bevacizumab
    (b) Cetuximab
    (c) Brentuximab
    (d) Ado-trastuzumab

    Answer: a

22. ONC201, being tried in the treatment of H3 K27M-mutant diffuse midline glioma, targets which receptor?

    (a) Dopamine
    (b) Glutamate
    (c) Glycine
    (d) Glutathione

    Answer: a

    ONC201 is a selective antagonist of dopamine receptor D2/3 (DRD2/3).

23. Which of the following is known as "tumor paint" and is a targeted fluorophore used in Fluorescent-Guided Surgery?

    (a) Indocyanine green
    (b) BLZ-100
    (c) Cetuximab-IRDye800
    (d) Alkyl Phosphocholine Analogs

    Answer: b

- BLZ-100 (Tozuleristide)—commonly known as "tumor paint"
- Conjugate of NIR with the tumor-specific peptide chlorotoxin
- Extracted from scorpion venom
- Chlorotoxin binds to the cell surface of low- and high-grade glial tumors
- Can be visualized with a NIR camera

24. Match the following subgroups of glioblastoma with their corresponding mutations.

(a) Proneural type	Neurofibromatosis type 1 (*NF1*) loss
(b) Mesenchymal type	Epidermal growth factor receptor (*EGFR*) amplifications and homozygous loss of *CDKN2A/B*
(c) Classical type	Cyclin-dependent kinase 4 (*CDK4*) and platelet-derived growth factor alpha (*PDGFRα*) amplification

Answer:

(a) Proneural type	Cyclin-dependent kinase 4 (CDK4) and platelet-derived growth factor alpha (PDGFRα) amplification
(b) Mesenchymal type	Neurofibromatosis type 1 (*NF1*) loss
(c) Classical type	Epidermal growth factor receptor (*EGFR*) amplifications and homozygous loss of *CDKN2A/B*

25. Match the following drugs being used in the trials for glioblastoma treatment with their corresponding mechanisms of action.

(a) Dichloroacetate	Tyrosine kinase inhibitor of MET
(b) Anhydrous enol-oxaloacetate	Inhibitor of tubulin polymerization
(c) Napabucasin	Produces glutamate scavenger
(d) Durvalumab (anti-CD274)	Glycolysis inhibitor
(e) Fuzuloparib	Prevents binding of PD-1 on PD-1 receptor
(f) Vorinostat	Proteasome inhibitor
(g) Marizomib	Histone deacetylase inhibitor
(h) Eribulin	Signal transducer and activator of transcription 2 (STAT3) inhibitor
(i) Cabozantinib	Induction of DNA double-strand breaks

Answer:

(a) Dichloroacetate	Glycolysis inhibitor
(b) Anhydrous enol-oxaloacetate	Produces glutamate scavenger
(c) Napabucasin	Signal transducer and activator of transcription 2 (STAT3) inhibitor
(d) Durvalumab (anti-CD274)	Prevents binding of PD-1 on PD-1 receptor
(e) Fuzuloparib	Induction of DNA double-strand breaks
(f) Vorinostat	Histone deacetylase inhibitor
(g) Marizomib	Proteasome inhibitor
(h) Eribulin	Inhibitor of tubulin polymerization
(i) Cabozantinib	Tyrosine kinase inhibitor of MET

26. Epithelioid glioblastomas are associated very frequently with a mutation in which of the following genes?

    (a) BRAF V600E
    (b) IDH 1
    (c) IDH 2
    (d) EGFR

    Answer: a

27. What is the usual location for chordoid glioma?

    (a) Temporal lobe
    (b) Anterior hypothalamus
    (c) Trigone
    (d) Occipital horn

    Answer: b

    Chordoid glioma—WHO grade 2
    Usually involves anterior third ventricle and hypothalamus

28. Which of the following is the most common gene fusion noted in glioblastoma?

    (a) Neurotrophic tyrosine receptor kinase (NTRK)
    (b) Fibroblast growth factor receptor (FGFR)
    (c) Mesenchymal-epithelial transition factor (MET)
    (d) Focal adhesion kinase (FAK)

    Answer: b

WHO Classification of Gliomas:

Adult-type diffuse gliomas
- Astrocytoma, IDH-mutant
- Oligodendroglioma, IDH-mutant, and 1p/19q-codeleted
- Glioblastoma, IDH-wildtype

Pediatric-type diffuse low-grade gliomas
- Diffuse astrocytoma, MYB- or MYBL1-altered
- Angiocentric glioma
- Polymorphous low-grade neuroepithelial tumor of the young
- Diffuse low-grade glioma, MAPK pathway-altered

Pediatric-type diffuse high-grade gliomas
- Diffuse midline glioma, H3 K27-altered
- Diffuse hemispheric glioma, H3 G34-mutant
- Diffuse pediatric-type high-grade glioma, H3-wildtype and IDH-wildtype
- Infant-type hemispheric glioma

Circumscribed astrocytic gliomas
- Pilocytic astrocytoma
- High-grade astrocytoma with piloid features
- Pleomorphic xanthoastrocytoma
- Subependymal giant cell astrocytoma
- Chordoid glioma
- Astroblastoma, MN1-altered

Test your learning and check your understanding of this book's contents: use the "Springer Nature Flashcards" app to access questions using https://sn.pub/3HwHCw To use the app, please follow the instructions in Chap. 1.

Bibliography

1. Oberheim-Bush NA, Shi W, McDermott MW, Grote A, Stindl J, Lustgarten L. The safety profile of Tumor Treating Fields (TTFields) therapy in glioblastoma patients with ventriculoperitoneal shunts. J Neuro-Oncol. 2022;158:453–61. https://doi.org/10.1007/s11060-022-04033-4.
2. Meena US, Sharma S, Chopra S, Jain SK. Gliosarcoma: a rare variant of glioblastoma multiforme in paediatric patient: case report and review of literature. World J Clin Cases. 2016;4(9):302–5. https://doi.org/10.12998/wjcc.v4.i9.302.
3. Wick W, Platten M, Weller M. New (alternative) temozolomide regimens for the treatment of glioma. Neuro-Oncology. 2009;11(1):69–79. https://doi.org/10.1215/15228517-2008-078.
4. Seo MJ, Lee DM, Kim IY, Lee D, Choi MK, Lee JY, Park SS, Jeong SY, Choi EK, Choi KS. Gambogic acid triggers vacuolization-associated cell death in cancer cells via disruption of thiol proteostasis. Cell Death Dis. 2019;10(3):187–16. https://doi.org/10.1038/s41419-019-1360-4.
5. Chen WL, Wagner J, Heugel N, Sugar J, Lee YW, Conant L, Malloy M, Heffernan J, Quirk B, Zinos A, Beardsley SA, Prost R, Whelan HT. Functional near-infrared spectroscopy and its clinical application in the field of neuroscience: advances and future directions. Front Neurosci. 2020;14:724. https://doi.org/10.3389/fnins.2020.00724.
6. Santosh V, Rao S. A review of adult-type diffuse gliomas in the WHO CNS5 classification with special reference to Astrocytoma, IDH-mutant and Oligodendroglioma, IDH-mutant and 1p/19q codeleted. Indian J Pathol Microbiol. 2022;65:S14–23. https://doi.org/10.4103/ijpm.ijpm_34_22.
7. Kunigelis KE, Vogelbaum MA. Therapeutic delivery to central nervous system. Neurosurg Clin N Am. 2021;32(2):291–303. https://doi.org/10.1016/j.nec.2020.12.004. Epub 2021 Feb 18
8. Bunevicius A, Sheehan JP. Radiosurgery for glioblastoma. Neurosurg Clin N Am. 2021;32(1):117–28. https://doi.org/10.1016/j.nec.2020.08.007. Epub 2020 Nov 5
9. Chi AS, Tarapore RS, Hall MD, Shonka N, Gardner S, Umemura Y, Sumrall A, Khatib Z, Mueller S, Kline C, Zaky W, Khatua S, Weathers SP, Odia Y, Niazi TN, Daghistani D, Cherrick I, Korones D, Karajannis MA, Kong XT, Minturn J, Waanders A, Arillaga-Romany I, Batchelor T, Wen PY, Merdinger K, Schalop L, Stogniew M, Allen JE, Oster W, Mehta MP. Pediatric and adult H3 K27M-mutant diffuse midline glioma treated with the selective DRD2 antagonist ONC201. J Neurooncol. 2019;145(1):97–105. https://doi.org/10.1007/s11060-019-03271-3. Epub 2019 Aug 27
10. Butte PV, Mamelak A, Parrish-Novak J, Drazin D, Shweikeh F, Gangalum PR, Chesnokova A, Ljubimova JY, Black K. Near-infrared imaging of brain tumors using the tumor paint BLZ-100

to achieve near-complete resection of brain tumors. Neurosurg Focus. 2014;36(2):E1. https://doi.org/10.3171/2013.11.FOCUS13497.

11. Melhem JM, Detsky J, Lim-Fat MJ, Perry JR. Updates in IDH-wildtype glioblastoma. Neurotherapeutics. 2022;31:1–19. https://doi.org/10.1007/s13311-022-01251-6. Epub ahead of print

12. Pająk B. Looking for the holy grail-drug candidates for glioblastoma Multiforme chemotherapy. Biomedicine. 2022;10(5):1001. https://doi.org/10.3390/biomedicines10051001.

13. Huang C, Gan D, Huang B, Luo J, Zhou X, Wang W, Wang Y. Chordoid glioma in the thalamus of a child: rare location and atypical imaging findings. BJR Case Rep. 2021;7(3):20200108. https://doi.org/10.1259/bjrcr.20200108.

14. Afonso M, Brito MA. Therapeutic options in neuro-oncology. Int J Mol Sci. 2022;23(10):5351. https://doi.org/10.3390/ijms23105351.

Chapter 16
Meningiomas

Joe M Das

1. DAL-1, a tumor suppressor gene identified in around 40% of sporadic meningiomas, is located in which chromosome?

    (a) 18p
    (b) 18q
    (c) 22p
    (d) 22q

    Answer: a

    The most common gene mutation in >50% of sporadic meningiomas—the NF2 gene (chromosome 22)

2. Match the following locations of meningiomas with their likely gene mutations.

(a) Anterior skull base	NF2
(b) Falx/parasagittal	SMARCE1
(c) Spinal meningioma in conjunction with cranial meningioma in a young patient	Smoothened (SMO) and v-akt murine thymoma viral oncogene homolog 1 (AKT1)

    Answer:

(a) Anterior skull base	Smoothened (SMO) and v-akt murine thymoma viral oncogene homolog 1 (AKT1)
(b) Falx/parasagittal	NF2
(c) Spinal meningioma in conjunction with cranial meningioma in a young patient	SMARCE1

J. M. Das (✉)
Consultant Neurosurgeon, Bahrain Specialist Hospital, Juffair, Bahrain
e-mail: neurosurgeon@doctors.org.uk

J. M. Das, *Neuro-Oncology Explained Through Multiple Choice Questions*,
https://doi.org/10.1007/978-3-031-13253-7_16

3. Which is not a feature of an atypical meningioma?

   (a) 4–19 mitotic figures in 10 consecutive high-powered fields (HPF)
   (b) 3 or more of 5 atypical features
   (c) Tumor invasion into brain
   (d) Predominant rhabdoid and papillary morphology

   Answer: d

   Atypical Features

   - Small cells with a high nuclear-to-cytoplasmic ratio
   - Increased cellularity
   - Prominent nucleoli
   - Sheet-like growth
   - Spontaneous necrosis

4. The loss of SMARCE1, resulting from SMARCE1 mutations, is pathognomonic for

   (a) Rhabdoid meningioma
   (b) Clear cell meningioma
   (c) Papillary meningioma
   (d) Chordoid meningioma

   Answer: b

   Chordoid and clear cell meningiomas—WHO grade 2.
   Rhabdoid and papillary meningioma—WHO grade 3.

5. Inactivation of the breast cancer BRCA1-associated protein (*BAP1*) or poly-
   bromo-1 (*PBRM1*) is associated with which of the following types of
   meningiomas?

   (a) Rhabdoid
   (b) Clear cell
   (c) Transitional
   (d) Chordoid

   Answer: a

6. Which of the following is not a feature of WHO grade 3 meningioma?

   (a) Homozygous loss of the tumor suppressor gene cyclin—dependent kinase
       inhibitor 2A/B (*CDKN2A/B*)
   (b) More than 19 mitotic figures in 10 consecutive HPFs
   (c) Mutations in the telomerase reverse transcriptase (*TERT*) gene promoter
   (d) Clear cell morphology

   Answer: d

7. Which statement is incorrect about the post-operative management of meningiomas?

(a) Small, asymptomatic recurrence of a WHO grade 1 meningioma does not warrant radiotherapy
(b) Radiotherapy has good local control rates if administered because of the progressive growth of a benign meningioma
(c) WHO grade 3 meningioma does not need adjuvant radiotherapy if the resection is complete
(d) Observation is suitable for WHO grade 2 meningiomas after complete resection

Answer: c

- Adjuvant radiotherapy is indicated in WHO grade 3 meningiomas regardless of the extent of resection.
- Radiotherapy has good local control rates of 92% at 15 years in benign meningiomas when administered due to:
  - Progressive growth or
  - Contraindication to surgical excision.

8. Which is a receptor tyrosine kinase inhibitor, with activity against VEGFR and platelet-derived growth factor receptor, being tried in the management of recurrent WHO grade 3 meningioma?

(a) Pasireotide
(b) Vismodegib
(c) Sunitinib
(d) Sandostatin

Answer: c

- Pasireotide, Sandostatin—Somatostatin analogs
- Vismodegib—SMO inhibitor

9. Which of the following is not a classification for posterior fossa meningiomas?

(a) Bradac
(b) Sekhar and Wright
(c) Castellano
(d) Sekhar-Mortazavi

Answer: d

10. Match the following classification systems with their corresponding location of meningiomas.

(a) Desgeorges and Sterkers classification	Tentorial notch
(b) Al-Mefty classification	Spine
(c) Bassiouni classification	Sphenoid wing

(d) Yasargil classification	Anterior midline skull base
(e) Brotchi and Pirotte classification	Posterior petrous
(f) Bayoumi classification	Falx meningioma
(g) Mohr classification	Tentorial
(h) Zuo classification	Clinoidal
(i) Sekhar-Mortazavi classification	Optic nerve sheath
(j) Shick classification	Planum sphenoidale and tuberculum sellae

Answer:

(a) Desgeorges and Sterkers classification	Posterior petrous
(b) Al-Mefty classification	Clinoidal
(c) Bassiouni classification	Tentorial notch
(d) Yasargil classification	Tentorial
(e) Brotchi and Pirotte classification	Sphenoid wing
(f) Bayoumi classification	Spine
(g) Mohr classification	Anterior midline skull base
(h) Zuo classification	Falx meningioma
(i) Sekhar-Mortazavi classification	Planum sphenoidale and tuberculum sellae
(j) Shick classification	Optic nerve sheath

11. Which of the following is not a classification of sinus invasion in parasagittal meningioma?

    (a) Sindou and Alvernia
    (b) Merrem-Krause
    (c) Bonnal-Brotchi
    (d) Dulguerov

    Answer: d

12. What are the contents in a Psammoma body?

    (a) Calcium apatite and elastin
    (b) Calcium apatite and collagen
    (c) Magnesium apatite and collagen
    (d) Magnesium apatite and elastin

    Answer: b

13. Modified Shinshu grade or Okudera-Kobayashi grade is used to denote

    (a) The grading of meningioma
    (b) The extent of resection of meningioma
    (c) The degree of brain invasion in a meningioma
    (d) The radiological response to adjuvant radiation therapy in a partially resected grade 2 meningioma

    Answer: b

14. Hirsch grading system is used to denote

(a) The degree of facial nerve involvement in cerebellopontine angle meningioma
(b) The encasement of cavernous carotid in cavernous sinus meningioma
(c) The encasement of the vertebral artery in foramen magnum meningioma
(d) The degree of abducens nerve involvement in falcotentorial meningioma

Answer: b

WHO Classification
Meningiomas • Meningioma

Mesenchymal, non-meningothelial tumors
•   Soft tissue tumors
    – Fibroblastic and myofibroblastic tumors
      Solitary fibrous tumor
    – Vascular tumors
      Hemangiomas and vascular malformations
      Hemangioblastoma
    – Skeletal muscle tumors
      Rhabdomyosarcoma
    – Uncertain differentiation
      Intracranial mesenchymal tumor, FET-CREB fusion-positive
      CIC-rearranged sarcoma
      Primary intracranial sarcoma, DICER1-mutant
      Ewing sarcoma

Melanocytic tumors
• Diffuse meningeal melanocytic neoplasms
    – Meningeal melanocytosis and meningeal melanomatosis
• Circumscribed meningeal melanocytic neoplasms
    – Meningeal melanocytoma and meningeal melanoma

Test your learning and check your understanding of this book's contents: use the "Springer Nature Flashcards" app to access questions using https://sn.pub/3HwHCw To use the app, please follow the instructions in Chap. 1.

Bibliography

1. McFaline-Figueroa JR, Kaley TJ, Dunn IF, Bi WL. Biology and treatment of Meningiomas: a reappraisal. Hematol Oncol Clin North Am. 2022;36(1):133–46. https://doi.org/10.1016/j.hoc.2021.09.003.

Chapter 17
Ependymal and Embryonal Tumors

Ryan M. Hess and Mohamed A. R. Soliman

17.1 Ependymal (Questions 1–12)

1. In the pediatric population, which of the following factors is associated with a reduced survival in regard to ependymoma?

   (a) Spinal location
   (b) Older age at diagnosis
   (c) Gross total resection
   (d) Diagnosis at younger than 3 years of age
   (e) Supratentorial location

   Answer: d

   The answer is younger age at diagnosis. Regarding survival, factors associated with an increased chance at survival include spinal location, older age at diagnosis, and gross total resection of the lesion. There is no difference in survival in patients with supratentorial lesions compared to infratentorial lesions in large population-based studies. Younger age at diagnosis is associated with

R. M. Hess
Department of Neurosurgery, Jacobs School of Medicine and Biomedical Sciences, University at Buffalo, Buffalo, NY, USA

Department of Neurosurgery, Buffalo General Medical Center, Kaleida Health, Buffalo, NY, USA

M. A. R. Soliman (✉)
Department of Neurosurgery, Faculty of Medicine, Cairo University, Cairo, Egypt
e-mail: moh.ar.sol@kasralainy.edu.eg

© The Author(s), under exclusive license to Springer Nature
Switzerland AG 2023
J. M. Das, *Neuro-Oncology Explained Through Multiple Choice Questions*,
https://doi.org/10.1007/978-3-031-13253-7_17

reduced chance of survival according to available data. Other important factors include extent of disease at diagnosis, histologic grade, and molecular subtype [1, 2].

2. The most common location for an ependymoma in the adult population is which location?

   (a) Lateral ventricle
   (b) Third ventricle
   (c) Floor of the fourth ventricle
   (d) Roof of the fourth ventricle
   (e) Ependyma of the central canal of the spinal cord

   Answer: e

   In adults, the most common location of an ependymoma is the ependyma of the central canal of the spinal cord. This contrasts with the pediatric population in which 80–90% of ependymomas arise intracranially [3].

3. Which of the following genetic alterations is most commonly seen in pediatric WHO Grade 2 or 3 ependymomas?

   (a) WNT
   (b) SHH
   (c) RELA fusion
   (d) 1p/19q co-deletion
   (e) INI1

   Answer: c

   The RELA fusion mutation has recently been identified as a key genetic mutation in >70% of supratentorial ependymomas in the pediatric population. Another commonly seen mutation in supratentorial ependymomas is the YAP-1 oncogene fusion. The WNT and SHH mutations are commonly seen in medulloblastomas. The 1p/19q co-deletion is associated with oligodendroglioma. Finally, INI1 mutations are most commonly seen in rhabdoid tumors [4–6].

4. Which of the following statements regarding the molecular subtypes of posterior fossa ependymomas is not true?

   (a) Group A tumors are associated with a worse prognosis
   (b) Group A tumors more commonly occur in a medial location
   (c) Group B tumors are associated with a more favorable prognosis
   (d) Group B tumors tend to occur in older patients with a median age of 20 years at diagnosis
   (e) Group A tumors tend to occur in a younger patient population with a median age of 2.5 years at diagnosis

   Answer: b

   Posterior fossa ependymomas can be sub-categorized based on gene profile and behavior into two groups: A and B. The A group is more laterally located, more aggressive, occurs in a younger population (median age of 2.5), has a higher risk of recurrence, and is associated with an overall poor prognosis. This is contrasted with the group B sub-classification which is seen in an older population of patients (median age of 20), is more medially located, are less aggressive, and are associated with a more favorable prognosis [7].

5. Which of the following ependymoma subtypes is classically located in the conus medullaris of an adult patient?

   (a) Subependymoma
   (b) Tanycytic
   (c) Clear cell
   (d) Myxopapillary
   (e) Anaplastic

   Answer: d

   Myxopapillary ependymomas are WHO Grade 1 ependymomas that are most commonly found in the conus medullaris in the adult population but can also be located within the cauda equina [8].

6. A 4-year-old child is brought to the emergency room by his mother for evaluation of progressive headaches and vomiting over the past 2 weeks. An MRI was performed which demonstrated a large posterior fossa mass. The patient was taken for surgical resection and the pathology is shown below:

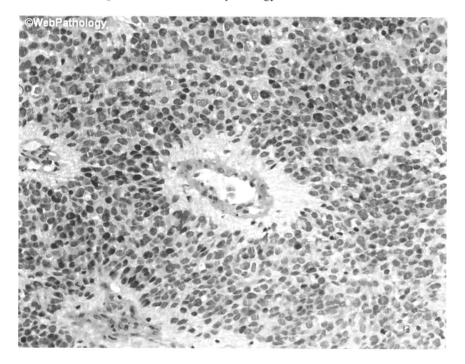

Based on the pathology slide, [9] which of the following diagnosis is most likely the daignosis?

(a) Medulloblastoma
(b) Ependymoma
(c) Meningioma
(d) Choroid plexus papilloma
(e) Astrocytoma

Answer: b

The above pathology slide demonstrates a perivascular pseudo-rosette, commonly seen in ependymoma specimens. The other answer choices typically do not have this finding on frozen section. Medulloblastoma can have a similar finding called a Homer-Wright rosette, however cells surround eosinophilic neuropil and not a blood vessel [10].

7. A five-year old female undergoes resection of a posterior fossa ependymoma found on work-up for progressive morning headaches. Gross total resection is achieved based upon post-operative MRI. Which of the following represents the most appropriate next step in the patient's treatment?

(a) Observation
(b) Chemotherapy alone
(c) Radiotherapy alone
(d) Chemotherapy and radiation therapy

Answer: c

Following surgical resection, post-operative radiotherapy plays an important role in the treatment of ependymomas. Studies have demonstrated improved rates of survival and local disease control in patients who undergo post-operative radiotherapy following resection. Unfortunately, the role of chemotherapy is not clear with current data not demonstrating a clear benefit of chemotherapy to the treatment paradigm [11–13].

8. Following surgical resection of an ependymoma, residual tumor greater than which threshold has been associated with a less favorable outcome?

(a) 0.5 cm^3
(b) 1 cm^3
(c) 1.5 cm^3
(d) 2 cm^3
(e) 2.5 cm^3

Answer: c

It has been shown that residual tumor burden following resection $>1.5 \text{ cm}^3$ has been associated with worse outcome in patients with the diagnosis of ependymoma [14].

9. Regarding ependymoma, which of the following factors is the most important determinant of outcome?

   (a) Extent at diagnosis
   (b) Location
   (c) Age at diagnosis
   (d) Extent of resection
   (e) Molecular classification

   Answer: d

   Though all the other answers are predictors of outcome, extent of surgical resection is the most important variable in determination of long-term prognosis in patients diagnosed with ependymoma. This has been demonstrated across several studies with survival rates being reported between 67–80% compared to 22–47% 5-year survival in patients with significant residual tumor burden [15–17].

10. Regarding the WHO classification of ependymoma subtypes, which of the following statements is true?

    (a) Papillary ependymomas are WHO grade 1 lesions
    (b) Pancytic ependymomas are WHO grade 3 lesions
    (c) Myxopapillary ependymomas are WHO grade 3 lesions
    (d) Subependymomas are WHO grade 1 lesions
    (e) Anaplastic ependymomas are WHO grade 1 lesions

    Answer: d

    Of the available answer choices, only C is correct. Subependymomas and Myxopapillary ependymomas are WHO grade 1. Tanycytic, papillary, and clear cell ependymomas are WHO grade 2. Anaplastic ependymomas are WHO grade 3 [8].

11. Patients with which of the following genetic conditions are predisposed to developing spinal ependymomas?

    (a) Neurofibromatosis I
    (b) Neurofibromatosis II
    (c) Gorlin Syndrome
    (d) Turcot Syndrome
    (e) Angelman Syndrome

    Answer: b

    Patients with neurofibromatosis type II have a genetic predisposition to develop spinal ependymomas due to the chromosomal mutation on chromosome 22 they harbor, as many ependymomas have mutations in chromosome 22 as well. However, it is likely that several areas of the chromosome are responsible for this predisposition as even patients without neurofibromatosis type II can have genetic mutations in chromosome 22 [18, 19].

12. Other than RELA mutations, what other genetic mutation is characteristic of pediatric supratentorial ependymomas?

  (a) Chromosome 22
  (b) INI1
  (c) YAP1
  (d) PTEN
  (e) P53

   Answer: c

   In addition to RELA mutations, the YAP1 mutation is characteristic of pediatric supratentorial ependymomas. The YAP1 protein is a downstream mediator of the tumor suppressing Hippo pathway [4, 20, 21].

17.2   Embryonal Tumors (Questions 1–13)

1. Based on the 2021 WHO Classification of Tumors of the Central Nervous system guidelines, which of the following is no longer considered to be a distinct pathologic entity?

  (a) Medulloblastoma
  (b) Atypical teratoid/rhabdoid tumors (AT/RT)
  (c) CNS neuroblastoma
  (d) Primitive neuroepithelial tumors (PNET)
  (e) CNS tumor with BCOR internal tandem duplication

   Answer: d

   In the current iteration of the WHO Classification of Tumors of the Central Nervous System, the term "PNET" was removed and replaced with embryonal tumors in order to reflect this version focus on molecular characterization. Broadly, embryonal tumors are poorly differentiated, hypercellular neoplasms that bear resemblance to the embryonic CNS, hence the name. In the past, tumors that had these characteristics on pathologic evaluation were labeled as PNETs, sometimes being subclassified based on location (medulloblastoma in posterior fossa for example). However, the ever-developing field of genomics has allowed for families of these tumors to be identified based on molecular subtypes. Currently, embryonal tumors include the following: medulloblastoma, AT/RT, CNS neuroblastoma, embryonal tumor with multilayered rosettes, CNS embryonal tumor not-otherwise specified, CNS tumor with BCOR internal tandem duplication, and cribriform neuroepithelial tumor [22].

2. A 2-year-old male is found to have a posterior fossa mass on work-up for increased lethargy and vomiting. The frozen specimen obtained during surgical resection is shown below. Based on the specimen, which diagnosis is most likely?

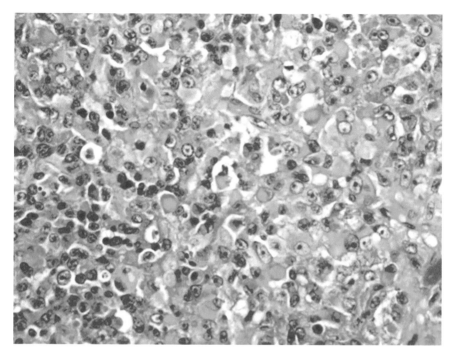

(a) AT/RT
(b) medulloblastoma
(c) ependymoma
(d) choroid plexus papilloma
(e) pilocytic astrocytoma

Answer: a

The Answer is AT/RT. The pathology slide shows classic histological findings of AT/RT which is the appearance of rhabdoid cells [23]. These cells are small and possess eccentric nuclei as well as globular eosinophilic inclusions. Mitotic figures are also common [24].

3. Which of the following mutations is most commonly associated with atypical teratoid/rhabdoid tumors?

(a) YAP1
(b) RELA
(c) KIAA1549-BRAF fusion
(d) SMARCB1 (INI1)
(e) Wnt

Answer: d

AT/RT is commonly associated with SMARCB1 (INI1) inactivation. It is occasionally associated inactivation of SMARCB4 as well. YAP1 and RELA are mutations associated with ependymomas. The KIAA1549-BRAF fusion is associated with pilocytic astrocytomas. Wnt mutations are commonly seen in medulloblastomas [25].

4. Outcome following diagnosis of an embryonal tumor is dictated by which of the following?

(a) Age at diagnosis
(b) Extent of surgical resection
(c) Presence of metastatic disease
(d) Only B and C
(e) All of the above

Answer: e

Age at diagnosis, extent of surgical resection, and presence of metastatic disease all influence outcome in patients diagnosed with embryonal tumors. Patients diagnosed younger than 3 years old, those with metastatic disease, and those with significant residual tumor volume following resection are more likely to have a poor outcome [26, 27].

5. Which of the following subgroups of embryonal tumors is not associated with alterations of C19MC microRNAs on chromosome 19?

(a) Ependymoblastoma
(b) Medulloepithelioma
(c) Embryonal tumor with abundant neuropil and true rosettes (ETANTR)
(d) Embryonal tumor with multilayered rosettes (ETMR)
(e) CNS neuroblastoma

Answer: e

The Answer is E. Answers A-D are currently considered to be under the ETMR C19MC sub-group of embryonal tumors due to all these entities having in common alterations of C19MC microRNAs on chromosome 19. Historically, these entities were considered separate diagnosis, however the recent iteration of WHO Classification of Tumors of the Central Nervous System has grouped them into one family of tumors due to the unifying presence of this mutation. This was done to better categorize an otherwise heterogeneously appearing group of tumors on pathology slides in order to better guide the development of treatment protocols [22, 28].

6. Which of the following is not considered one of the four main molecular subtypes of medulloblastoma?

(a) Wnt
(b) SHH
(c) Group 3
(d) YAP1
(e) Group 4

Answer: d

The four main molecular subtypes of medulloblastoma are Wnt, SHH, group 3, and group 4. Proper identification of the subtype through molecular testing is critical for treatment and determining prognosis, as each group behaves as its own pathologic entity. YAP1 is a mutation associated with some forms of ependymoma [29].

7. Which of the four molecular subtypes of medulloblastoma has the best prognosis?

   (a) Wnt
   (b) SHH
   (c) Group 3
   (d) Group 4

   Answer: a

   Of the four subtypes of medulloblastoma, Wnt has the best prognosis while group 3 has the worst prognosis [30].

8. Which of the following is the most common subtype of medulloblastoma?

   (a) Group 3
   (b) Group 4
   (c) Wnt
   (d) SHH
   (e) RELA

   Answer: b

   Group 4 medulloblastoma is the most common, accounting for 35% of cases. The Wnt subtype is the least common, accounting only for 10% of medulloblastoma cases [30].

9. Which genetic abnormality seen in the group 3 subtype of medulloblastoma is associated with the worst prognosis?

   (a) SMARCA4
   (b) GFI1
   (c) Isochromosome 17q
   (d) KBTDB4
   (e) MYC

   Answer: e

   Unlike the Wnt and SHH subtypes of medulloblastoma, the group 3 subtype is not defined by abnormalities in a specified signaling pathway. Instead, it is a heterogenous group composed of tumors with similar underlying behavior and genetic abnormalities. Group 3 medulloblastomas can be subcategorized into 3 alpha, 3 beta, and 3 gamma. Group 3 gamma is associated with mutations in the MYC gene and has the worse prognosis of any group 3 medulloblastoma. 5-year survival is only 41% [31].

10. In patients with medulloblastoma, residual tumor volume greater than what threshold has been associated with worse outcome?

  (a) 0.5 cm^3
  (b) 1.0 cm^3
  (c) 1.5 cm^3
  (d) 2.0 cm^3
  (e) 2.5 cm^3

  Answer: c

  Patients with medulloblastoma with residual tumor burden of $>1.5 \text{ cm}^3$ following surgical resection have been shown to have lower odds of survival and reduced progression free survival [32].

11. Which of the following statements regarding post-operative adjuvant radiotherapy in patients with medulloblastoma is most accurate?

  (a) Chemotherapy is commonly deferred in children younger than three until recurrence or until they reach the age of three
  (b) All patients older than 3 years receive 36 Gy of craniospinal irradiation followed by a boost to 54 Gy to the posterior fossa regardless of molecular subtype
  (c) There are attempts to limit radiation dose in patients older than 3 years of age with low risk or average risk medulloblastoma by using chemotherapeutics during radiotherapy treatments
  (d) A and C
  (e) A and B

  Answer: c

  Currently, there have been several attempts to use the molecular classification schemes in order to modify treatment regimens for patients with medulloblastoma. Radiotherapy is a good example of this given its association with delayed toxicity. As such, irradiating all patients with the previous standard 36 Gy of craniospinal irradiation followed by a boost to 54 Gy to the posterior fossa is becoming less common. There is evidence suggesting that patients with low or average risk medulloblastoma have favorable outcomes with reduced radiation dosing if chemotherapy is given along with it. However, high risk patients with aggressive forms of medulloblastoma continue to receive the standard dosage regimen of radiation. Similarly, recent data has shown favorable outcomes in patients younger than 3 years of age if they are treated first with chemotherapy and radiation is deferred until they are older than 3 or there is recurrence [33–35].

12. Which of the following clinical features of medulloblastoma are associated with poor outcome?

  (a) Age younger than 3 at the age of diagnosis
  (b) Residual tumor $>1.5 \text{cm}^3$ after resection

(c) Leptomeningeal spread at diagnosis
(d) Only A and C
(e) All of the above

Answer: e

Age younger than 3 at diagnosis, residual tumor >1.5 cm^3, and leptomeningeal spread are all clinical features associated with poor prognosis in patients with medulloblastoma. Patients with these characteristics have traditionally been termed "high-risk" [36, 37].

13. A 6-year-old male is diagnosed with a posterior fossa mass after presenting to the emergency room with 1 month of morning headaches. He is taken for surgical resection and the patient is found to have the SHH variant of medulloblastoma. Broadly speaking, which of the following answer choices best characterizes his adjuvant treatment?

(a) No adjuvant treatment, only observation is recommended
(b) Chemotherapy with a combination of cisplatin, carboplatin, and vincristine only
(c) 36 Gy of craniospinal irradiation followed by a boost to 54 Gy to the posterior fossa only
(d) Chemotherapy with need for and dosing of craniospinal irradiation based on risk
(e) Stereotactic radiosurgery to the resection bed followed by an inhibitor of the SHH signaling pathway

Answer: d

In general, adjuvant chemotherapy followed by risk-based radiotherapy is the standard treatment following surgical resection in patients with medulloblastoma. The importance of molecular subtypes is highlighted by this treatment paradigm, as patients with less aggressive subtypes, such as Wnt, may be treated successfully with chemotherapy only, or receive radiotherapy in a reduced dose. Other less fortunate patients with metastatic disease at presentation or high-risk subtypes, like group 3, require aggressive craniospinal irradiation in addition to chemotherapy. At this time, there is not a clear role for stereotactic radiosurgery in the treatment of medulloblastoma, though it has been used as salvage therapy in recurrent disease. Finally, advanced biologics that target specific signaling mediators are not yet widely available. Additionally, large clinical trials demonstrating their benefit are not yet available but are currently being conducted [33, 38–41].

WHO Classification of Ependymal Tumors

Supratentorial ependymoma
- Supratentorial ependymoma, ZFTA fusion-positive
- Supratentorial ependymoma, YAP1 fusion-positive

Posterior fossa ependymoma
- Posterior fossa ependymoma, group PFA
- Posterior fossa ependymoma, group PFB

Spinal ependymoma
- Spinal ependymoma, MYCN-amplified
- Myxopapillary ependymoma
- Subependymoma

WHO Classification of Embryonal Tumors

Medulloblastoma
- Medulloblastomas, molecularly defined
  - Medulloblastoma, WNT-activated
  - Medulloblastoma, SHH-activated and TP53-wildtype
  - Medulloblastoma, SHH-activated and TP53-mutant
  - Medulloblastoma, non-WNT/non-SHH
- Medulloblastomas, histologically defined

Other CNS embryonal tumors
- Atypical teratoid/rhabdoid tumor
- Cribriform neuroepithelial tumor
- Embryonal tumor with multilayered rosettes
- CNS neuroblastoma, FOXR2-activated
- CNS tumor with BCOR internal tandem duplication
- CNS embryonal tumor

Image attributions:

1. WebPathology
2. Nirupama Singh, M.D., Ph.D., and PathologyOutlines.com.

Test your learning and check your understanding of this book's contents: use the "Springer Nature Flashcards" app to access questions using https://sn.pub/3HwHCw To use the app, please follow the instructions in Chap. 1.

References

1. Cage TA, Clark AJ, Aranda D, et al. A systematic review of treatment outcomes in pediatric patients with intracranial ependymomas. J Neurosurg Pediatr. 2013;11:673–81.
2. McGuire CS, Sainani KL, Fisher PG. Both location and age predict survival in ependymoma: a SEER study. Pediatr Blood Cancer. 2009;52:65–9.
3. Villano JL, Parker CK, Dolecek TA. Descriptive epidemiology of ependymal tumours in the United States. Br J Cancer. 2013;108:2367–71.
4. Pajtler KW, Pfister SM, Kool M. Molecular dissection of ependymomas. Oncoscience. 2015;2:827–8.

5. Pietsch T, Wohlers I, Goschzik T, et al. Supratentorial ependymomas of childhood carry C11orf95-RELA fusions leading to pathological activation of the NF-kappaB signaling pathway. Acta Neuropathol. 2014;127:609–11.
6. Pajtler KW, Witt H, Sill M, et al. Molecular classification of ependymal tumors across all CNS compartments, histopathological grades, and age groups. Cancer Cell. 2015;27:728–43.
7. Witt H, Mack SC, Ryzhova M, et al. Delineation of two clinically and molecularly distinct subgroups of posterior fossa ependymoma. Cancer Cell. 2011;20:143–57.
8. International Agency for Research on Cancer (IARC). WHO classification of Tumours of the central nervous system. 4th ed. Lyon: IARC; 2016.
9. Webpathology.com (image).
10. Godfraind C. Classification and controversies in pathology of ependymomas. Childs Nerv Syst. 2009;25:1185–93.
11. Merchant TE, Li C, Xiong X, et al. Conformal radiotherapy after surgery for paediatric ependymoma: a prospective study. Lancet Oncol. 2009;10:258–66.
12. Merchant TE, Haida T, Wang MH, et al. Anaplastic ependymoma: treatment of pediatric patients with or without craniospinal radiation therapy. J Neurosurg. 1997;86:943–9.
13. Chiu JK, Woo SY, Ater J, et al. Intracranial ependymoma in children: analysis of prognostic factors. J Neuro Oncol. 1992;13:283–90.
14. Robertson PL, Zeltzer PM, Boyett JM, et al. Survival and prognostic factors following radiation therapy and chemotherapy for ependymomas in children: a report of the Children's Cancer Group. J Neurosurg. 1998;88:695–703.
15. Foreman NK, Love S, Thorne R. Intracranial ependymomas: analysis of prognostic factors in a population-based series. Pediatr Neurosurg. 1996;24:119–25.
16. Sutton LN, Goldwein J, Perilongo G, et al. Prognostic factors in childhood ependymomas. Pediatr Neurosurg. 1990;16:57–65.
17. Healey EA, Barnes PD, Kupsky WJ, et al. The prognostic significance of postoperative residual tumor in ependymoma. Neurosurgery. 1991;28:666–71. discussion 671–672
18. Wernicke C, Thiel G, Lozanova T, et. al. Involvement of chromosome 22 in ependymomas. Cancer Genet Cytogenet. 1995;79:173–6.
19. Ebert C, von Haken M, Meyer-Puttlitz B, et. al. Molecular genetic analysis of ependymal tumors. NF2 mutations and chromosome 22q loss occur preferentially in intramedullary spinal ependymomas. Am J Pathol. 1999;155:627–32.
20. Parker M, Mohankumar KM, Punchihewa C, et al. C11orf95-RELA fusions drive oncogenic NF-kappaB signalling in ependymoma. Nature. 2014;506:451–5.
21. Andreiuolo F, Varlet P, Tauziede-Espariat A, et. al. Childhood supratentorial ependymomas with YAP1-MAMLD1 fusion: an entity with characteristic clinical, radiological, cytogenetic and histopathological features. Brain Pathol. 2019;29:205–16.
22. Louis DN, Perry A, Wesseling P, Brat DJ, Cree IA, Figarella-Branger D, Hawkins C, Ng HK, Pfister SM, Reifenberger G, Soffietti R, von Deimling A, Ellison DW. The 2021 WHO classification of tumors of the central nervous system: a summary. Neuro-Oncology. 2021;23(8):1231–51.
23. https://www.pathologyoutlines.com/topic/cnstumoratypicalteratoidrhabdoid.html. Accessed May 4th, 2022. (image).
24. Biegel JA. Molecular genetics of atypical teratoid/rhabdoid tumor. Neurosurg Focus. 2006;20:E11.
25. Ho B, Johann PD, Grabovska Y, et al. Molecular subgrouping of atypical teratoid/rhabdoid tumors-a reinvestigation and current consensus. Neuro-Oncology. 2020;22:613–24.
26. Albright AL, Wisoff JH, Zeltzer P, et al. Prognostic factors in children with supratentorial (non-pineal) primitive neuroectodermal tumors. A neurosurgical perspective from the Children's Cancer Group. Pediatr Neurosurg. 1995;22:1–7.
27. Hong TS, Mehta MP, Boyett JM, et al. Patterns of failure in supratentorial primitive neuroectodermal tumors treated in Children's Cancer Group Study 921, a phase III combined modality study. Int J Radiat Oncol Biol Phys. 2004;60:204–13.

28. Korshunov A, Sturm D, Ryzhova M, et al. Embryonal tumor with abundant neuropil and true rosettes (ETANTR), ependymoblastoma, and medulloepithelioma share molecular similarity and comprise a single clinicopathological entity. Acta Neuropathol. 2014;128:279–89.
29. Northcott PA, Korshunov A, Witt H, et al. Medulloblastoma comprises four distinct molecular variants. J Clin Oncol. 2011;29:1408–14.
30. Juraschka K, Taylor MD. Medulloblastoma in the age of molecular subgroups: a review. J Neurosurg Pediatr. 2019;24(4):353–63.
31. Cavalli FMG, Remke M, Rampasek L, et. al. Intertumoral heterogeneity within medulloblastoma subgroups. Canc Cell. 2017;31:737–54. e6.
32. Thompson EM, Bramall A, Herndon JE, Taylor MD, Ramaswamy V. The clinical importance of medulloblastoma extent of resection: a systematic review. J Neuro Oncol 2018;139:523–39.
33. Gajjar A, Chintagumpala M, Ashley D, et al. Risk-adapted craniospinal radiotherapy followed by high-dose chemotherapy and stem-cell rescue in children with newly diagnosed medulloblastoma (St Jude Medulloblastoma-96): long-term results from a prospective, multicentre trial. Lancet Oncol. 2006;7:813–20.
34. Oyharcabal-Bourden V, Kalifa C, Gentet JC, et al. Standard-risk medulloblastoma treated by adjuvant chemotherapy followed by reduced-dose craniospinal radiation therapy: a French society of pediatric oncology study. J Clin Oncol. 2005;23:4726–34.
35. Jakacki RI, Feldman H, Jamison C, Boaz JC, Luerssen TG, Timmerman R. A pilot study of preirradiation chemotherapy and 1800 cGy craniospinal irradiation in young children with medulloblastoma. Int J Radiat Oncol Biol Phys. 2004;60:531–6.
36. Packer RJ, Cogen P, Vezina G, et al. Medulloblastoma: clinical and biologic aspects. Neuro Oncol 1999;1:232–50.
37. Packer RJ, Vezina G: Management of and prognosis with medulloblastoma: therapy at a crossroads. Arch Neurol. 2008;65:1419–24.
38. Packer RJ, Gajjar A, Vezina G, et al. Phase III study of craniospinal radiation therapy followed by adjuvant chemotherapy for newly diagnosed average-risk medulloblastoma. J Clin Oncol. 2006;24:4202–8.
39. Gandola L, Massimino M, Cefalo G, et al. Hyperfractionated accelerated radiotherapy in the milan strategy for metastatic medulloblastoma. J Clin Oncol. 2009;27:566–71.
40. Zhao M, Wang X, Fu X, Zhang Z. Bevacizumab and stereotactic radiosurgery achieved complete response for pediatric recurrent medulloblastoma. J Cancer Res Ther. 2018;14: S789–S792.
41. St. Jude Children's Research Hospital. A clinical and molecular risk-directed therapy for newly diagnosed medulloblastoma. ClinicalTrials.gov. 2021.

Chapter 18
Pituitary and Sellar Tumors

Ahmed A. Najjar and Mohammed Jawhari

1. Which of the following is the most common type of metastatic tumors to the sellar region in men?

   (a) Liver
   (b) Lung
   (c) Prostate
   (d) Colon

   Answer: b

   Lung and breast cancers are the most common types of cancers in both sexes. Prostate cancer does not usually give distant metastases to the sellar region. Liver cancer usually spreads to the lungs and bones. Colon cancer metastasis to the brain is also very rare and indicates a very aggressive disease.

2. Which of the following is the most common type of metastatic tumors to the sellar region in women?

   (a) Breast
   (b) Ovaries
   (c) Uterus
   (d) Lung

   Answer: a

A. A. Najjar (✉)
College of Medicine, Taibah University, Medina, Saudi Arabia
e-mail: anajjar@taibahu.edu.sa

M. Jawhari
Neurosurgery Resident, King Fahad General Hospital, Medina, Saudi Arabia

© The Author(s), under exclusive license to Springer Nature Switzerland AG 2023
J. M. Das, *Neuro-Oncology Explained Through Multiple Choice Questions*,
https://doi.org/10.1007/978-3-031-13253-7_18

177

Breast cancer is the most common source of brain metastases in females. Lung cancer is also common but not as common as breast cancer in females. Uterine and ovarian cancer metastasize the brain but much less frequently.

3. All the following anatomical structures can be a source of sellar extension of a meningioma except

(a) Tuberculum sellae
(b) Dorsum sellae
(c) Diaphragma sellae
(d) Olfactory grove

Answer: d

Meningiomas of the sellar region can arise from adjacent structures. Olfactory groove meningiomas usually need to be very large to reach the sellar area but they don't most of the time. The sellar area is subject to invasion from adjacent structures commonly tuberculum sellae, planum sphenoidal, diaphragma sellae, anterior clinoid, cavernous sinus, and dorsum sellae.

4. Which of the following is the most typical histological feature found in granular cell tumors of the pituitary stalk?

(a) PAS positive granules
(b) High Ki-67 index
(c) Beta Catenin
(d) EMA

Answer: a

Granular cell tumor of the pituitary stalk is a rare entity. The most typical feature is the abundance of periodic acid-Schiff granules in the ample cytoplasm. Typically, it is a benign tumor. Beta-catenin and epithelial membrane antigen (EMA) are positive for craniopharyngiomas.

5. Which of the following is the most common subtype of functioning pituitary adenoma?

(a) Prolactinoma
(b) Acromegaly
(c) Cushing disease
(d) TSH-producing pituitary adenoma

Answer: a

Pituitary neuroendocrine tumors (PitNETs) and pituitary adenomas are very common. Prolactinoma is the most common functioning subtype. TSH-secreting adenomas are the least common type.

6. Factors affecting the recurrence of pituitary adenomas include all the following except

   (a) Tumor size
   (b) Post-operative residue
   (c) Invasive tumor
   (d) Post-operative radiotherapy

   Answer: d

   Pituitary adenomas are very common. Treatment usually is effective. Factors that affect recurrence include the size of the tumor, preoperative hormone levels, invasiveness of the tumor, and younger age. Post-operative radiotherapy is associated with a lower recurrence rate.

7. The histologic feature predicting the metastatic potential of pituitary adenomas includes

   (a) P53
   (b) Ki-67
   (c) Cell type
   (d) Mitotic activity

   Answer: d

   There is no World Health Organization (WHO) grade for pituitary adenomas according to the 2017 classification. The use of P53 and Ki-67 alone for grading is largely abandoned. The concept of lineage-specific classification was introduced. Pituitary adenomas should be assessed according to their proliferation (mitotic count and Ki-67 indices), tumor invasiveness, and functional status.

8. After resection of a pituitary adenoma, histology shows the presence of large dysmorphic ganglionic cells that are positive for neuronal markers and negative for glial markers. What is the histologic diagnosis?

   (a) Pleurihormonal PIT-1 positive adenoma
   (b) Ganglioglioma
   (c) Mixed Pituitary Adenoma-Gangliocytoma
   (d) Prolactinoma

   Answer: c

   Mixed Pituitary Adenoma- Gangliocytoma is a rare tumor. It represents the neuronal metaplasia of adenoma cells. Usually, it is reactive to neuronal markers and negative for glial markers. They can be positive for pituitary hormones.

9. A 53-year-old lady, known to have Hashimoto thyroiditis, presents with an enhancing sellar mass. You decided to operate. Histology shows lymphocytic heavy infiltration. Which is the following is the most likely diagnosis?

   (a) Pituitary adenoma
   (b) Hypophysitis

(c) Lymphoma
(d) Pituiticytoma

Answer: b

Hypophysitis is a rare mimicker to pituitary tumors. There is usually a history of autoimmune disease or the use of checkpoint inhibitors or other targeted therapies. Histopathology confirms the diagnosis. The prognosis generally depends on the cause with primary hypophysitis having a bit better prognosis than secondary hypophysitis.

10. Differential diagnoses of a sellar cystic mass include all of the following except

(a) Rathke cleft cyst
(b) Arachnoid cyst
(c) Meningioma
(d) Epidermoid cyst

Answer: c

Cystic sellar and suprasellar masses are common. Meningioma is usually solid in sellar and suprasellar region. Rathke pouch and arachnoid cysts are developmental in origin. Epidermoid cyst can be mistaken for a Rathke pouch cyst and may need histopathology to distinguish between the two entities.

11. Which of the following histologic markers is a hallmark of pituicytomas?

(a) Galectin-3
(b) TTF-1
(c) PIT-1
(d) EMA

Answer: b

Pituicytomas arise from the posterior hypophysis. TTF-1 positivity is a characteristic feature of tumors of posterior hypophysis origin. Galactin-3 is not positive in pituicytomas as well as PIT-1. EMA is positive for epithelial tumors.

12. Which of the following histological appearances is suggestive of brain invasion in adamantinomatous craniopharyngioma?

(a) Dense nodules and trabeculae of squamous epithelium bordered by a palisade of columnar epithelium
(b) Yellow-brown, cholesterol-rich fluid
(c) The presence of an isolated nest of tumor cells surrounding brain tissue
(d) Well-differentiated surface epithelium lacking surface maturation

Answer: c

Admantinomatous craniopharyngioma is a distinct histopathological entity. Pathologically, they are characterized by dense nodules and trabeculae of squamous epithelium bordered by columnar epithelium. The cystic part contains yellow-brown cholesterol-rich fluid. On the other hand, the papillary type is rarely cystic and has well-differentiated surface epithelium lacking maturation. Invasiveness criteria are controversial but having brain tissue surrounded by tumor cells isolated from the rest of the tumor is an accepted criterion to define invasiveness.

13. A 45-year-old male came to your clinic complaining of erectile dysfunction. He is generally healthy and has been with the same partner for the last 15 years. You order labs that come back as showing normal prolactin, low luteinizing hormone and follicle-stimulating hormone, and very low testosterone, with normal thyroid-stimulating hormone. What is the next step?

(a) Prescribe a low dose of sildenafil
(b) Order an MRI brain with IV contrast
(c) Reassure and educate
(d) Prescribe testosterone

Answer: b

Hypogonadotropic hypogonadism is associated with very low levels of testosterone (less than 150 ng/dl). Usually, the MRI of the brain will reveal a tumor in the pituitary gland. Prescribing a low dose of sildenafil at this stage is not helpful. Testosterone might help, but it is not the first step. Gonadotropin-releasing hormone hypo-functioning adenomas can affect also other hormones in the anterior pituitary.

14. The most sensitive test to detect visual field defects in patients with pituitary adenoma is

(a) Fundoscopy
(b) Central visual field test
(c) Peripheral visual field test
(d) Slit-lamp examination

Answer: c

Visual field defects are common in cases of macroadenomas. Peripheral visual field testing is the most sensitive test to detect defects. Central visual field tests are less sensitive as the compression is usually on the optic chiasm. Slit-lamp examination is not used for visual field testing.

15. Regarding Atypical Teratoid/Rhabdoid Tumor (AT/RT), which of the following is true?

(a) It is common in adults
(b) It is usually a benign tumor
(c) Leptomeningeal dissemination is common in pediatrics
(d) Usually positive for GFAP and IDH1 mutation

Answer: c

AT/RT is a rare type of brain tumor in adults. It is a malignant tumor most commonly in children younger than 3 years. Leptomeningeal metastasis is common in children, up to 25%. It is diagnosed histologically by loss of INI-1 or BRG1 proteins or genetic alterations in the SMARCB1 or SMARC4A genes.

16. A 13-year-old boy presents with a headache, visual defects, and imbalance for the past few weeks. CT and MRI brain revealed the presence of hydrocephalus as well as sellar and pineal region masses. A preliminary diagnosis of germ cell tumor is made. Surgery was done and a biopsy was taken from the pineal lesion that confirmed the diagnosis of germinoma. What is true regarding germinoma?

   (a) Isochromosome 12p is commonly seen
   (b) It is morphologically distinct from seminoma
   (c) The treatment of choice is surgery
   (d) The most common presenting symptom is diabetes insipidus

   Answer: d

   Intracranial germ cell tumors including germinoma represent 5% of intracranial lesions. They are morphologically similar to seminomas. Though isochromosome 12p is a characteristic of seminoma, it is rarely present in intracranial germinoma. The treatment is usually radiation therapy and surgery alone is not curative.

17. For pituitary apoplexy which of the following is the most sensitive MRI sequence for infarcted pituitary?

   (a) T1- weighted imaging with gadolinium
   (b) T2-weighted images
   (c) Diffusion-weighted images (DWI)
   (d) Gradient echo sequences (GRE)

   Answer: c

   Diffusion-weighted imaging is very useful to document pituitary infarction in ischemic (non-hemorrhagic) apoplexy. It demonstrates the infarcted area within a few minutes of arterial compromise. T1 with gadolinium is used for enhancing lesions like tumors. GRE is sensitive to blood products and is not the first choice for ischemia. T2-weighted images are not used to detect pituitary infarction.

18. Regarding outcomes of endoscopic endonasal surgery (EES) for large pituitary adenomas, which statement is true?

   (a) Cavernous sinus invasion, large size, intraventricular extension, and firm consistency were significant factors in determining the extent of resection (EoR)
   (b) Redo-surgery in 50% of cases
   (c) CSF leak happens in 50% of the cases
   (d) Radiotherapy is needed in more than 30% of cases

   Answer: a

EES is very effective and nowadays becoming more frequently used for large pituitary adenomas. The rate of gross total resection is 50% of the cases. Factors affecting the extent of resection include the size, degree of invasion of the adjacent structures, and tumor-related factors. Redo surgery occurs only in about 3% of the cases. CSF leak occurs in 10–20% of the cases. Radiotherapy is needed in only 5% of treated cases.

19. Regarding sellar and suprasellar dermoid and epidermoid cysts, which statement is true?

   (a) The most common location is in the sella
   (b) They are treated medically
   (c) Epidermoid is usually midline and dermoid is off midline
   (d) Surgical treatment, when indicated, is the mainstay of management

   Answer: d

   Dermoid and epidermoid lesions are rare intracranial pathologies that are rarely purely sellar. They usually extend to the sella from suprasellar or rarely sphenoidal locations. Dermoid is usually midline while epidermoid is off midline. Surgery remains the main form of therapy when indicated with a recurrence of up to 26%.

20. Which of the following is the most common pituitary tumor in McCune-Albright syndrome?

   (a) GH-secreting adenomas
   (b) Prolactinomas
   (c) TSH-secreting adenomas
   (d) Nonfunctioning adenomas

   Answer: a

   McCune-Albright syndrome (MAS) is a rare genetic disease. It has the triad of polyostotic fibrous dysplasia, precocious puberty, and café-au-lait spots. It is caused by a post-zygotic spontaneous mutation of the GNAS gene. GH-secreting adenomas are the most common. Other types of adenomas typically do not occur in MAS. The prognosis is worse than in isolated cases.

21. All of the following are considered a syndromic familial pituitary adenoma except

   (a) MEN 1
   (b) MEN 4
   (c) USP8-related syndrome
   (d) FIPA

   Answer: d

   Familial Pituitary Adenomas are of two kinds: syndromic or isolated. Isolated familial pituitary adenomas (FIPA) are less common and they usually occur in younger patients. The mutation is in the aryl hydrocarbon receptor-interacting protein (AIP) gene. The other 3 options are syndromic having pituitary adenomas plus other body tumors. Multiple Endocrine Neoplasia 1 and 4 are associated with MEN1 and MEN 4 mutations, respectively. Ubiquitin-specific peptidase 8 gene mutations predispose to delayed development of pituitary adenomas, dysmorphic features as well as lung disease.

22. Regarding sellar glomus tumors, which statement is true?

    (a) They are common
    (b) They can be easily diagnosed with the help of an MRI
    (c) They are classified as benign, of uncertain malignancy, or malignant
    (d) The treatment of choice is medical

    Answer: c

    Sellar glomus tumors are very rare mesenchymal tumors. They can be easily misdiagnosed as pituitary adenoma. The MRI is not specific. Histologically, they are classified as benign, of uncertain malignancy, or malignant based on nuclear atypia and mitosis. The treatment of choice is complete surgical resection.

23. Craniopharyngioma can be treated successfully with all of the following except

    (a) BRAF-V600E- inhibitors like dabrafenib and trametinib
    (b) Temozolomide
    (c) Interferon-a
    (d) Bleomycin

    Answer: b

    Papillary and adamantinomatous types of craniopharyngiomas are distinct histopathologies. BRAF-V600E mutation-positive tumors can be successfully treated with BRAF-V600E- inhibitors. Interferon-alfa is used very successfully for the cysts associated with adamantinomatous craniopharyngiomas. Bleomycin is used in the same way as interferon but with more toxicity. Temozolomide is not a medical treatment for craniopharyngiomas. It is mainly used for malignant gliomas.

24. The most sensitive pituitary adenoma to gamma knife therapy is

    (a) Prolactinoma
    (b) ACTH-secreting adenomas
    (c) Non-functioning pituitary adenoma
    (d) Growth hormone (GH)-secreting adenoma

    Answer: c

    Gamma Knife radiation therapy has been used successfully in the treatment of pituitary adenomas. With appropriate size, non-functioning tumors respond the most to radiation. Prolactinomas respond the least with about 50% achieving remission. Other functioning adenomas have a response rate of 60%.

25. The following are correct matches of immunohistochemical markers for pituitary tumors except

    (a) PIT-1: Somatotrophs, lactotrophs, and thyrotrophs
    (b) T-PIT: Corticotrophs
    (c) SF-1: Gonadotrophs
    (d) TIFF-1: Germ cells

    Answer: d

    TIFF-1 is an immunohistochemical marker that is useful to differentiate tumors originating from the pituitary gland from metastases. It is positive in pulmonary and some extrapulmonary tumors. All other matches are correct, and they must be done for each case of pituitary adenomas.

26. Which is true concerning the medical management of Cushing disease?

    (a) Has no role
    (b) Surgery is curative in 100% of cases
    (c) Retinoic acid, gefitinib, and seliciclib are new treatments
    (d) Dopamine agonists work effectively

    Answer: c

    Cushing disease is caused by pituitary adenomas primarily secreting ACTH. Surgery is still not curative in a large proportion of patients. New medical therapies directly targeting ACTH and cortisol secretion such as retinoic acid provide promise. Gefitinib and seliciclib are anti-EGFR and anti-CDK, respectively. Clinical trials are undergoing assessing their effectiveness. Dopamine agonists are used for prolactinomas and are not frequently used for Cushing disease.

27. With the 2017 WHO new classification of endocrine tumors, silent corticotroph adenomas (SCA) were introduced as a new entity. Which is true regarding this new entity?

    (a) It is introduced as a subtype of functioning adenomas
    (b) They are reportedly aggressive and highly invasive
    (c) Low-risk tumors
    (d) They are positive for PIT-1

    Answer: b

    SCA is introduced as a new entity in the 2017 WHO classification of endocrine tumors. They are a subtype of non-functioning pituitary adenomas. They are usually aggressive and highly invasive, so they were classified as high risk in the WHO classification. They are of corticotroph lineage positive for T-PIT, T BOX family member. PIT-1 is for cells of somatotroph, lactotroph, and thyrotroph lineage.

28. The true statement regarding pituitary stalk interruption syndrome is

    (a) Triad of ectopic posterior pituitary tissue, thin or absent pituitary stalk, and hypoplastic anterior pituitary
    (b) SIADH, syndrome of inappropriate ADH secretion, is the main presenting feature
    (c) Symptoms are due to the anterior hypophysis
    (d) It is a common radiological finding

    Answer: a

    Pituitary stalk interruption syndrome is a very rare disease. It is characterized by hypoplasia of the anterior hypophysis, thin or absent stalk, and ectopic posterior pituitary near the lamina terminalis. It presents with central diabetes insipidus in 10% of cases. The treatment is symptomatic.

29. Differential diagnosis of pituitary carcinoma includes all of the following except

    (a) Aggressive pituitary adenoma
    (b) Renal cell carcinoma
    (c) Multiple myeloma
    (d) Colon cancer

    Answer: d

    Primary pituitary carcinoma is very rare. It is necessary to have distant metastasis with histological resemblance to the primary tumor to make the diagnosis. There is no histological criteria to differentiate it from aggressive pituitary adenomas. It can resemble many cancers. Chromogranin-A and synaptophysin are useful to distinguish the origin of the tumor.

30. All of the following are complications of the transsphenoidal approach except

    (a) Internal carotid artery injury
    (b) New cranial nerve palsy
    (c) Cerebrospinal fluid leak
    (d) Seizure

    Answer: d

    Transsphenoidal surgery for pituitary, sellar, and suprasellar lesions is becoming the standard surgical approach. Internal carotid artery injury occurs in about 2% of cases and is a very serious occurrence. New cranial nerve palsy occurs in 7% of the cases. CSF leak occurs in about 5% of the cases. Seizure is not known to happen as a direct complication of the transsphenoidal approach.

WHO Classification of Tumors of the Sellar Region

- Adamantinomatous craniopharyngioma
- Papillary craniopharyngioma
- Pituicytoma, granular cell tumor of the sellar region, and spindle cell oncocytoma
- Pituitary adenoma/PitNET
- Pituitary blastoma

Test your learning and check your understanding of this book's contents: use the "Springer Nature Flashcards" app to access questions using https://sn.pub/3HwHCw To use the app, please follow the instructions in Chap. 1.

Bibliography

1. Abad AP. Sellar and Parasellar pain syndromes. Curr Pain Headache Rep. 2019;23:7.
2. Albano L, Losa M, Barzaghi LR, et al. Gamma knife radiosurgery for pituitary tumors: a systematic review and meta-analysis. Cancers (Basel). 2021;13:4998.
3. Altay T, Krisht KM, Couldwell WT. Sellar and parasellar metastatic tumors. Int J Surg Oncol. 2012;2012:647256.
4. Barry S, Korbonits M. Update on the genetics of pituitary tumors. Endocrinol Metab Clin N Am. 2020;49:433–52.
5. Bogusławska A, Gilis-Januszewska A, Korbonits M. Genetics of pituitary adenomas. In: Tamagno G, Gahete MD, editors. Pituitary adenomas: the European neuroendocrine Association's young researcher committee overview. Cham: Springer International Publishing; 2022. p. 83–125.
6. Burcea I, Poiana C. Updates in aggressive pituitary tumors. Acta Endocrinol (Buchar). 2020;16:267–73.
7. Cheng Y, Tang H, Wu ZB. Sellar Glomus tumor misdiagnosed as pituitary adenoma: a case report and review of the literature. Front Endocrinol (Lausanne). 2022;13:895054.
8. Chibbaro S, Signorelli F, Milani D, et al. Primary endoscopic Endonasal Management of Giant Pituitary Adenomas: outcome and pitfalls from a large prospective multicenter experience. Cancers (Basel). 2021;13:3603.
9. Fetcko K, Dey M. Primary central nervous system germ cell tumors: a review and update. Med Res Arch. 2018;6(3):1719.
10. Gregoire A, Bosschaert P, Godfraind C. Granular cell tumor of the pituitary stalk: a rare and benign entity. J Belg Soc Radiol. 2015;99:79–81.
11. Jiang S, Chen X, Wu Y, Wang R, Bao X. An update on silent Corticotroph adenomas: diagnosis, mechanisms, clinical features, and management. Cancers (Basel). 2021;13
12. Lara-Velazquez M, Mehkri Y, Panther E, et al. Current advances in the management of adult craniopharyngiomas. Curr Oncol. 2022;29:1645–71.
13. Li Z, Liu R, Liu P. McCune-Albright syndrome associated with pituitary adenoma: a clinicopathological study of ten cases and literature review. Br J Neurosurg. 2021:1–10.
14. Lu L, Wan X, Xu Y, Chen J, Shu K, Lei T. Prognostic factors for recurrence in pituitary adenomas: recent Progress and future directions. Diagnostics (Basel). 2022;12:977.
15. Nussbaum PE, Nussbaum LA, Torok CM, Patel PD, Yesavage TA, Nussbaum ES. Case report and literature review of BRAF-V600 inhibitors for treatment of papillary craniopharyngiomas: a potential treatment paradigm shift. J Clin Pharm Ther. 2022;47(6):826–31.
16. Ouyang T, Zhang N, Xie S, et al. Outcomes and complications of aggressive resection strategy for pituitary adenomas in Knosp grade 4 with Transsphenoidal endoscopy. Front Oncol. 2021;11:693063.
17. Raverot G, Burman P, McCormack A, et al. European Society of Endocrinology Clinical Practice Guidelines for the management of aggressive pituitary tumours and carcinomas. Eur J Endocrinol. 2018;178:G1–G24.
18. Sahakian N, Castinetti F, Brue T, Cuny T. Current and emerging medical therapies in pituitary tumors. J Clin Med. 2022;11:PMC8877616.
19. Schwetye KE, Dahiya SM. Sellar tumors. Surg Pathol Clin. 2020;13:305–29.
20. Tavakol S, Catalino MP, Cote DJ, Boles X, Laws ER Jr, Bi WL. Cyst type differentiates Rathke cleft cysts from cystic pituitary adenomas. Front Oncol. 2021;11:778824.

21. Tena-Suck ML, Hernández-Campos ME, Plataa AO, Sánchez-Garibay C, Salinas Lara C, Peñafiel C. Craniopharyngioma brain invasion forms. International Journal of Pathology and Clinical Research. 2019;5:94.
22. Varlamov EV, McCartney S, Fleseriu M. Functioning pituitary adenomas - current treatment options and emerging medical therapies. Eur Endocrinol. 2019;15:30–40.
23. Voellger B, Zhang Z, Benzel J, et al. Targeting aggressive pituitary adenomas at the molecular level-a review. J Clin Med. 2021;11:124.
24. Zada G, Lopes MBS, Mukundan S, Laws E. Sellar region epidermoid and dermoid cysts. In: Zada G, Lopes MBS, Mukundan Jr S, Laws Jr ER, editors. Atlas of sellar and parasellar lesions: clinical, radiologic, and pathologic correlations. Cham: Springer International Publishing; 2016. p. 245–50.

Chapter 19
Pineal Region Tumors

Joe M Das

1. Which of the following structures is located ventral to the pineal gland?

    (a) Corpus callosum
    (b) Habenular commissure
    (c) Posterior commissure
    (d) Superior cerebellar cistern

    Answer: c

    The Relations of the Pineal Gland are

    • Ventral—posterior commissure
    • Superior—corpus callosum
    • Dorsal—habenular commissure
    • Postero-inferior—Superior cerebellar cistern

2. Which of the following blood vessels does not provide blood supply to the pineal gland?

    (a) Medial choroidal arteries
    (b) Lateral choroidal arteries
    (c) Pericallosal artery
    (d) Posterior communicating artery

    Answer: d

    The arterial supply to the pineal gland is by

    • Medial choroidal artery
    • Lateral choroidal artery

J. M. Das (✉)
Consultant Neurosurgeon, Bahrain Specialist Hospital, Juffair, Bahrain
e-mail: neurosurgeon@doctors.org.uk

© The Author(s), under exclusive license to Springer Nature
Switzerland AG 2023
J. M. Das, *Neuro-Oncology Explained Through Multiple Choice Questions*,
https://doi.org/10.1007/978-3-031-13253-7_19

The anastomoses supplying these vessels are formed by

- Pericallosal arteries
- Posterior cerebral arteries
- Superior cerebellar arteries
- Quadrigeminal arteries

3. Which of the following tumors in the pineal region is likely to displace the deep venous system structures ventrally and inferiorly?

   (a) Germinoma
   (b) Teratoma
   (c) Velum interpositum meningioma
   (d) Pineocytoma

   Answer: c

   - Pineal tumors usually displace the deep venous system structures superiorly, except:

       – Velum interpositum meningiomas
       – Epidermoid or other tumors originating in the corpus callosum
   - The latter two displace the venous structures ventrally and inferiorly.

4. Which is the most aggressive form of gestational trophoblastic disease?

   (a) Pineal choriocarcinoma
   (b) Pineal teratoma
   (c) Pineal germinoma
   (d) Pineal embryonal carcinoma

   Answer: a

5. A 30-year-old lady presents with headaches and an MRI scan of the head shows a lesion in the pineal region without hydrocephalus. Her serum alfa-feto protein levels are high. What is the next step in the management of this patient?

   (a) Surgical resection
   (b) Endoscopic third ventriculostomy and biopsy
   (c) Stereotactic needle biopsy
   (d) Chemo/radiotherapy

   Answer: d

   - The patient is having the diagnosis of an endodermal sinus tumor, as the alfa-feto protein levels are high - which is pathognomonic.
   - Since she is not having hydrocephalus, ETV is not indicated.
   - Biopsy is not needed in this condition as the serum markers are high, which is quite diagnostic.
   - Pineal region tumors that should be treated based on high tumor marker levels and without a tissue diagnosis—nongerminomatous malignant germ cell tumors.

- These include:
  - Endodermal sinus tumors
  - Choriocarcinomas
  - Embryonal carcinomas

6. Which of the following are the second most common pineal tumors?

   (a) Germinomas
   (b) Choriocarcinomas
   (c) Teratomas
   (d) Pineal parenchymal tumors

   Answer: c

   The most common pineal gland neoplasms—Germ Cell Tumors (GCT) (60%)—include **germinoma, mature/immature teratoma**, embryonal carcinoma, yolk sac tumor, choriocarcinoma, and mixed GCT.

   The next common pineal gland tumor is PPT (half as common as the GCT).

7. Which surgical approach is suitable for tumors that extend inferiorly into the quadrigeminal plate?

   (a) Supracerebellar infratentorial
   (b) Occipital transtentorial
   (c) Interhemispheric transcallosal
   (d) b or c

   Answer: d

   Either the occipital transtentorial or the interhemispheric transcallosal approach is preferable in the following conditions:

   - Tumors that extend superiorly, involving or destroying the posterior aspect of the corpus callosum and deflecting the deep venous system in a dorsolateral direction
   - Tumors that extend laterally to the region of the trigone
   - Tumors that extend inferiorly into the quadrigeminal plate
   - In rare cases in which the tumor displaces the deep venous system in a ventral direction

8. Lateral Supracerebellar Infratentorial approach is over the surface of which lobule of the cerebellum?

   (a) Gracile
   (b) Quadrangular
   (c) Biventral
   (d) Semilunar

   Answer: b

9. What is the initial line of management for a 5-year-old child with pineoblastoma?

   (a) Biopsy
   (b) Surgery
   (c) Chemotherapy
   (d) Radiotherapy

   Answer: b

   - **The initial line of management for children ≤3 years:**
     Biopsy followed by chemotherapy
   - **The initial line of management for children >3 years:**
     Surgery followed by adjuvant radiotherapy ± adjuvant chemotherapy

10. What is the common mutation found in the desmoplastic myxoid tumor of the pineal region?

    (a) SMARCB1
    (b) SMARCB2
    (c) SMARCB3
    (d) SMARCB4

    Answer: a

    Desmoplastic myxoid tumor (DMT), SMARCB1-mutant

    - Recently proposed brain tumor.
    - Occurs in the pineal region of adults.
    - Characterized by desmoplastic stroma and various degrees of a myxoid matrix.

11. Which of the following statements regarding pineal tumor markers is false?

    (a) Embryonal carcinomas, immature teratomas, and endodermal sinus tumors can cause elevated AFP
    (b) Choriocarcinomas and germinomas can be associated with elevated β-hCG
    (c) Germinomas with elevated β-hCG may have a good prognosis.
    (d) Germinomas can be associated with elevated LDH and pALP

    Answer: c

    - Germinomas associated with elevated β-hCG may have a poor prognosis.
    - Mature teratomas tend to be negative for serum and cerebrospinal fluid alpha-fetoprotein.

12. The standard treatment for pineal parenchymal tumors is

    (a) Surgery
    (b) Radiation
    (c) Chemotherapy
    (d) Chemoradiation

    Answer: b

13. The most common initial symptom of a pineal tumor is

    (a) Headache
    (b) Diplopia
    (c) Upgaze palsy
    (d) Day-time somnolence

    Answer: a

    • Headache is usually due to hydrocephalus occurring secondary to aque-
      ductal compression.

14. Which of the following is not seen in Parinaud syndrome?

    (a) Lid retraction
    (b) Convergence-retraction nystagmus
    (c) Light-near pupillary dissociation
    (d) Downgaze paralysis

    Answer: d

    The classical features of Parinaud syndrome are:

    • Paralysis of upgaze
    • Convergence-retraction nystagmus
    • Light-near pupillary dissociation
    • Dorsal midbrain compression → lid retraction (the Collier sign) or ptosis.

    Further midbrain compression → Sylvian aqueduct syndrome → paralysis of
    downgaze/horizontal gaze from further midbrain compression.

15. What is the cell of origin of the papillary tumor of the pineal region?

    (a) Ependyma of the third ventricle
    (b) Ependyma of subcommissural organ
    (c) Choroid plexus papillae
    (d) Capillary cells in the medial choroidal artery

    Answer: b

16. Spinal MRI to look for spinal seeding is not required for patients with which of
    the following tumors?

    (a) Pineal cell tumors
    (b) Malignant germ cell tumors
    (c) Ependymomas
    (d) Germinomas

    Answer: d

17. What is the most common site of origin of metastasis in the pineal region?

    (a) Lung
    (b) Breast

(c) Prostate
(d) Pancreas

Answer: a

18. Which is a novel marker useful for the grading and prognostic evaluation of pineal parenchymal tumors of intermediate differentiation?

(a) CD4
(b) CD24
(c) CD44
(d) CD144

Answer: b

CD24 and PRAME are novel markers for pineal parenchymal tumors of intermediate differentiation.

WHO classification of pineal tumors

- Pineocytoma
- Pineal parenchymal tumor of intermediate differentiation
- Pineoblastoma
- Papillary tumor of the pineal region
- Desmoplastic myxoid tumor of the pineal region, SMARCB1-mutant

WHO classification of germ cell tumors

- Mature teratoma
- Immature teratoma
- Teratoma with somatic-type malignancy
- Germinoma
- Embryonal carcinoma
- Yolk sac tumor
- Choriocarcinoma
- Mixed germ cell tumor

Test your learning and check your understanding of this book's contents: use the "Springer Nature Flashcards" app to access questions using https://sn.pub/3HwHCw To use the app, please follow the instructions in Chap. 1.

Bibliography

1. Favero G, Bonomini F, Rezzani R. Pineal gland tumors: a review. Cancers (Basel). 2021;13(7):1547. https://doi.org/10.3390/cancers13071547.
2. Vuong HG, Ngo TNM, Dunn IF. Incidence, prognostic factors, and survival trend in pineal gland tumors: a population-based analysis. Front Oncol. 2021;19(11):780173. https://doi.org/10.3389/fonc.2021.780173.

3. Childhood Medulloblastoma and Other Central Nervous System Embryonal Tumors Treatment (PDQ®).
4. Matsumura N, Goda N, Yashige K, Kitagawa M, Yamazaki T, Nobusawa S, Yokoo H. Desmoplastic myxoid tumor, SMARCB1-mutant: a new variant of SMARCB1-deficient tumor of the central nervous system preferentially arising in the pineal region. Virchows Arch. 2021;479(4):835–9. https://doi.org/10.1007/s00428-020-02978-3. Epub 2021 Jan 9
5. Carr C, O'Neill BE, Hochhalter CB, Strong MJ, Ware ML. Biomarkers of pineal region tumors: a review. Ochsner J. 2019;19(1):26–31. https://doi.org/10.31486/toj.18.0110.
6. Li J, Recinos PF, Orr BA, Burger PC, Jallo GI, Recinos VR. Papillary tumor of the pineal region in a 15-month-old boy. J Neurosurg Pediatr. 2011;7(5):534–8. https://doi.org/10.317 1/2011.2.PEDS10434.
7. Alaminus G, Frappaz D, Kortmann RD, Krefeld B, Saran F, Pietsch T, Vasiljevic A, Garre ML, Ricardi U, Mann JR, Göbel U, Alapetite C, Murray MJ, Nicholson JC. Outcome of patients with intracranial non-germinomatous germ cell tumors-lessons from the SIOP-CNS-GCT-96 trial. Neuro-Oncology. 2017;19(12):1661–72. https://doi.org/10.1093/neuonc/nox122.
8. Wu X, Wang W, Lai X, Zhou Y, Zhou X, Li J, Liang Y, Zhu X, Ren X, Ding Y, et al. CD24 and PRAME are novel grading and prognostic indicators for pineal parenchymal tumors of intermediate differentiation. Am J Surg Pathol. 2020;44:11–20. https://doi.org/10.1097/PAS.0000000000001350.

Chapter 20
Vestibular Schwannoma

Joe M Das

1. Which is the most common extra-axial posterior fossa tumor in adults?

   (a) Meningioma
   (b) Metastasis
   (c) Vestibular schwannoma
   (d) Osteoma

   Answer: c

2. What is the most common presentation of a patient with vestibular schwannoma?

   (a) Unilateral sensorineural hearing loss
   (b) Tinnitus
   (c) Vertigo
   (d) Unsteadiness

   Answer: a

3. Which is not a heavily T2-weighted MRI sequence used to evaluate the vestibulocochlear nerve and its branches in relation to a vestibular schwannoma?

   (a) FIESTA
   (b) CISS
   (c) DRIVE
   (d) PROPELLER

   Answer: d

   • FIESTA—Fast Imaging Employing Steady-state Acquisition
   • CISS—Constructive Interference in Steady State

J. M. Das (✉)
Consultant Neurosurgeon, Bahrain Specialist Hospital, Juffair, Bahrain
e-mail: neurosurgeon@doctors.org.uk

J. M. Das, *Neuro-Oncology Explained Through Multiple Choice Questions*,
https://doi.org/10.1007/978-3-031-13253-7_20

- DRIVE—Driven equilibrium pulse
- PROPELLER—Periodically Rotated Overlapping Parallel lines with Enhanced Reconstruction—used to reduce motion artifact in T2-weighted images

4. Which of the following statements is false regarding the variants of vestibular schwannomas?

   (a) Cellular schwannoma is characterized by the predominance of Antoni A pattern and absence of properly formed Verocay bodies
   (b) Melanotic schwannoma expresses HMB45
   (c) There is a 10% risk for malignant transformation in melanotic schwannoma
   (d) Psammomatous melanotic schwannoma is always associated with the Carney complex

   Answer: d

   - Psammomatous melanotic schwannoma has a 50% association with the Carney complex.
   - Melanotic schwannomas are associated with mutations ins GNAQ/GNA11, BRAF, and pTERT.

5. A vestibular schwannoma protruding into the cerebellopontine angle but not touching the brain stem belongs to which Koos grade?

   (a) I
   (b) II
   (c) III
   (d) IV

   Answer: b

   - Grade 1: Small intracanalicular tumor
   - Grade II: Tumor protruding into the cerebellopontine angle but not touching the brain stem (<2 cm)
   - Grade III: Tumor occupying CP angle cistern with no displacement of the brainstem (<3 cm)
   - Grade IV: Brainstem and cranial nerve displacement (>3 cm)

6. Which is not a factor that influences the preservation of serviceable hearing after microsurgery?

   (a) Tumor size <1 cm
   (b) Presence of distal internal auditory canal CSF fundal cap
   (c) Good preoperative hearing function
   (d) Age < 80 years

   Answer: d

7. What is the dose of radiation used in stereotactic radiosurgery for vestibular schwannoma?

   (a) 6–10 Gy
   (b) 11–14 Gy
   (c) 15–20 Gy
   (d) 21–24 Gy

   Answer: b

8. The maximum threshold dose of radiation at the modiolus of the cochlea reported for functional hearing preservation is

   (a) 1 Gy
   (b) 2 Gy
   (c) 3 Gy
   (d) 4 Gy

   Answer: d

9. What is the only known environmental risk factor for sporadic vestibular schwannoma?

   (a) High-dose ionizing radiation
   (b) Use of mobile phone
   (c) Ebstein-Barr Virus infection
   (d) Ramsay-Hunt syndrome

   Answer: a

10. Which drug is used in the treatment of neurofibromatosis type 2 patients with progressive vestibular schwannomas?

    (a) Bebtelovimab
    (b) Bevacizumab
    (c) Tixagevimab
    (d) Cilgavimab

    Answer: b

11. What is the treatment of choice for a patient with a small vestibular schwannoma with impaired hearing?

    (a) Observation
    (b) Stereotactic radiosurgery
    (c) Retrosigmoid approach and tumor resection
    (d) Translabyrinthine approach and tumor resection

    Answer: b

    - Symptomatic small tumor with impaired hearing (Koos grade I-II) is managed better with SRS as it provides a lower risk of facial paresis compared to surgery

12. What is the definition of serviceable hearing?

    (a) Pure-tone average of ≥50 dB and a speech discrimination score of ≤50%
    (b) Pure-tone average of ≤25 dB and a speech discrimination score of ≥75%
    (c) Pure-tone average of ≤ 50 dB and a speech discrimination score of ≥ 50%
    (d) Pure-tone average of ≥25 dB and a speech discrimination score of ≤75%

    Answer: c

    "Good" hearing is defined as a speech discrimination score of 70% or greater.

13. Which are the most important waves in BAER while performing surgery on vestibular schwannoma?

    (a) Acoustic nerve, Superior olives, Inferior colliculi
    (b) Acoustic nerve, Lateral lemniscus, Inferior colliculi
    (c) Cochlear nuclei, Superior olives, Inferior colliculi
    (d) Cochlear nuclei, Lateral lemniscus, Medial geniculate body

    Answer: a

    Wave I—Acoustic nerve
    Wave II—Cochlear nuclei
    Wave III—Superior olives
    Wave IV—Lateral lemniscus tracts and nuclei
    Wave V—Inferior colliculi
    Waves VI—Medial geniculate body
    Wave VII— Auditory radiations to the temporal lobe
    Waves I, III, and V are the most important ones during intraoperative monitoring.

14. The most common location of the facial nerve in relation to a vestibular schwannoma is

    (a) Anterosuperiorly
    (b) Anteroinferiorly
    (c) Posterosuperiorly
    (d) Posteroinferiorly

    Answer: a

15. What are the anterior and posterior limits of drilling the internal auditory canal?

    (a) Anterior limit—Trigeminal ganglion; posterior limit—Glasscock's triangle
    (b) Anterior limit—Kawase's triangle; posterior limit—Arcuate eminence
    (c) Anterior limit—Trigeminal ganglion, posterior limit—Kawase's triangle
    (d) Anterior limit—Foramen spinosum, posterior limit—Arcuate eminence

    Answer: b

16. Which is not a poor prognostic factor for hearing preservation during vestibular schwannoma surgery?

   (a) Abnormal ABR Latency
   (b) Inferior vestibular nerve origin
   (c) Superior vestibular nerve origin
   (d) Opacification of the fundus of the internal auditory canal by tumor

   Answer: c

   • Poor prognostic signs for hearing preservation include the following:

   – Abnormal auditory brainstem response latency
   – Inferior vestibular nerve origin
   – Fundus opacification by the tumor

17. Changes to the latency or amplitude of the which cochlear nerve action potential (CNAP) wave peak suggests neural injury while performing vestibular schwannoma surgery?

   (a) P1
   (b) P2
   (c) N1
   (d) N2

   Answer: c

   WHO classification of cranial and paraspinal nerve tumors

• Schwannoma
• Neurofibroma
• Perineurioma
• Hybrid nerve sheath tumor
• Malignant melanotic nerve sheath tumor
• Malignant peripheral nerve sheath tumor
• Paraganglioma

Test your learning and check your understanding of this book's contents: use the "Springer Nature Flashcards" app to access questions using https://sn.pub/3HwHCw To use the app, please follow the instructions in Chap. 1.

Bibliography

1. Goldbrunner R, Weller M, Regis J, Lund-Johansen M, Stavrinou P, Reuss D, Evans DG, Lefranc F, Sallabanda K, Falini A, Axon P, Sterkers O, Fariselli L, Wick W, Tonn JC. EANO guideline on the diagnosis and treatment of vestibular schwannoma. Neuro-Oncology. 2020;22(1):31–45. https://doi.org/10.1093/neuonc/noz153.

2. Mohindra N, Neyaz Z. Magnetic resonance sequences: practical neurological applications. Neurol India. 2015;63(2):241–9. https://doi.org/10.4103/0028-3886.156293.
3. Sartoretti-Schefer S, Kollias S, Valavanis A. Spatial relationship between vestibular schwannoma and facial nerve on three-dimensional T2-weighted fast spin-echo MR images. AJNR Am J Neuroradiol. 2000;21(5):810–6.
4. Hoa M, Drazin D, Hanna G, Schwartz MS, Lekovic GP. The approach to the patient with incidentally diagnosed vestibular schwannoma. Neurosurg Focus. 2012;33(3):E2. https://doi.org/10.3171/2012.6.FOCUS12209.

Chapter 21
Intraventricular Tumors

Joe M Das

1. The venous angle is formed between

    (a) Anterior septal vein and thalamostriate vein
    (b) Thalamostriate vein and internal cerebral vein
    (c) Anterior septal vein and internal cerebral vein
    (d) Thalamostriate vein and thalamocaudal vein

   Answer: b

   - The U-shaped angle at the junction of the thalamostriate and internal cerebral veins—venous angle
   - Anatomic landmark for access to the third ventricle via the lateral ventricle.
   - True venous angle is adjacent to the posterior margin of the foramen of Monro.
   - False venous angle lies behind it.
   - The location of the anterior septal vein (ASV)–internal cerebral vein (ICV) junction determines the limit of posterior enlargement of the foramen of Monro.
   - An ASV terminating at the ICV at the venous angle → disadvantage for surgical exposure
   - An ASV joining the trunk of the ICV → advantage for surgical exposure
   - Türe et al., subclassified the true (type I) and false (type II) venous angles further into subtypes:

       - A, in which the ASV–ICV junction is located at the venous angle
       - B, in which the ASV joins the main stem of the ICV beyond the venous angle.

J. M. Das (✉)
Consultant Neurosurgeon, Bahrain Specialist Hospital, Juffair, Bahrain
e-mail: neurosurgeon@doctors.org.uk

© The Author(s), under exclusive license to Springer Nature Switzerland AG 2023
J. M. Das, *Neuro-Oncology Explained Through Multiple Choice Questions*,
https://doi.org/10.1007/978-3-031-13253-7_21

- 4 venous angle types (IA, IB, IIA, IIB).
- Typically, this junction is located 3 to 7 mm posterior to the foramen of Monro.

2. The inferior choroidal point is located at which edge of the uncus?

(a) Anterosuperior
(b) Posterosuperior
(c) Anteroinferior
(d) Posteroinferior

Answer: b

- The anterior choroidal artery enters the choroidal fissure at the inferior choroidal point.
- Located at the posterosuperior edge of the uncus and anterior limit of the body of the hippocampus.
- Represents the inferolateral end of the choroidal fissure.
- The anterior choroidal artery enters the choroidal fissure at the inferior choroidal point.
- Foramen of Monro corresponds to the superior choroidal point.

3. Which statement is false regarding velum interpositum?

(a) It is a space between the two layers of the tela choroidea in the roof of the third ventricle
(b) The contents include the internal cerebral veins and their tributaries and lateral posterior choroidal arteries
(c) The space above the velum interpositum between the hippocampal commissure and splenium is called the cavum vergae
(d) It may have an opening situated between the splenium and pineal body that communicates with the quadrigeminal cistern to form the velum interpositum cistern.

Answer: b

The contents include the internal cerebral veins and their tributaries and medial posterior choroidal arteries.

4. If a patient is noted to have right homonymous hemianopsia with macular sparing preoperatively, extensive damage to the splenium during a posterior interhemispheric transcallosal approach results in

(a) Alexia with agraphia
(b) Alexia without agraphia
(c) Agraphia without alexia
(d) Color agnosia

Answer: b

5. The supracerebellar transtentorial approach to the ventricular atrium is done via the

    (a) Collateral sulcus
    (b) Occipitotemporal sulcus
    (c) Calcarine sulcus
    (d) Rhinal sulcus

    Answer: a

6. Which is not a structure forming the roof of the third ventricle?

    (a) Fornix
    (b) Choroid plexus
    (c) Velum interpositum
    (d) Thalamus

    Answer: d

    The roof of the third ventricle is formed by:

    • Fornices
    • Superior membrane of the tela choroidea
    • Velum interpositum (containing the internal cerebral veins and medial posterior choroidal artery)
    • Inferior membrane of the tela choroidea
    • Third ventricular choroid plexus

7. Posterior third ventricle is difficult to be accessed via which of the following approaches?

    (a) Transforaminal transchoroidal
    (b) Transforaminal subchoroidal
    (c) Transforaminal
    (d) Interforniceal

    Answer: c

8. Which is the most accurate variable for determining the prognosis of central neurocytoma?

    (a) MIB-1 labeling index
    (b) Mitotic index
    (c) Degree of positive staining for NeuN
    (d) The presence of Oligodendrocyte transcription factor 2 (Olig2)

    Answer: a

    Olig2 is generally absent in central neurocytoma, but present in oligodendroglioma.

9. What is the most common location of a central neurocytoma?

   (a) Frontal horn of right lateral ventricle
   (b) Frontal horn of left lateral ventricle
   (c) Body of right lateral ventricle
   (d) Body of left lateral ventricle

   Answer: b

   • The majority of ventricular meningiomas are located in the lateral ventricle atrium—left side.
   • Most choroid plexus papillomas are located in the lateral ventricle atrium (left > right) in pediatric patients. In adults, a fourth ventricular location is the most common.
   • Ependymomas arise anywhere within the ventricular system with a predilection for the fourth ventricle, especially in pediatric patients.

10. Which is a sensitive and specific marker for choroid plexus papilloma?

   (a) Stanniocalcin-1
   (b) CD7
   (c) CD20
   (d) Microtubule-associated protein

   Answer: a

   • Both sensitive and specific—Kir7.1 and stanniocalcin-1
   • CK7+/CD20−—to differentiate choroid plexus tumor from metastatic tumor
   • Choroid plexus tumors—positive for E-cadherin and negative for NCAM
   • Ependymomas-negative for E-cadherin and positive for NCAM.
   • PTPRs can be distinguished from choroid plexus tumors by their expression of microtubule-associated protein 2 and NCAM.
   • The most common underlying genetic mechanism identified in choroid plexus carcinomas is TP53 dysfunction.

11. Which is not a component of the colloid cyst risk score?

   (a) Age
   (b) Axial diameter
   (c) FLAIR hyperintensity
   (d) Presence of hydrocephalus

   Answer: d

Criterion	Points	
Age < 65 years	Yes-1	No-0
Headache	Yes-1	No-0
Axial diameter ≥ 7 mm	Yes-1	No-0
FLAIR hyperintensity	Yes-1	No-0
Risk zone	Yes-1	No-0

- Zone 1: Extending from the lamina terminalis posteriorly to a tangent line between the mammillary bodies and the anterior aspect of the mass intermedia. Cysts in zone 1 are considered at risk of occluding the foramen of Monro.
- Zone 2: Extending from the posterior aspect of zone 1 to the anterior border of the cerebral aqueduct. Cysts in zone 2 are considered at low risk of obstructing CSF flow.
- Zone 3: Extends from the posterior aspect of zone 2 to the posterior border of the third ventricle. Cysts in zone 3 are considered at risk of occluding the cerebral aqueduct.

    A colloid cyst risk score of ≥4 is high risk and associated with obstructive hydrocephalus, while a score ≤ 2 represents a low-risk group.

12. Which radiological feature is present in both colloid cyst and Rathke cleft cyst?

    (a) T2 dot sign
    (b) Polka dot sign
    (c) Murphy sign
    (d) Salmon patch sign

    Answer: a

13. What is the most common type of intraventricular meningioma?

    (a) Transitional
    (b) Fibrous
    (c) Meningothelial
    (d) Psammomatous

    Answer: b

14. A newborn baby is noted to have anorectal malformation, sacral agenesis, and a doubtful epidermoid tumor in the presacral region. What is the most common mutation associated with this condition?

    (a) DLK1
    (b) GLK1
    (c) MEN1
    (d) MNX1

    Answer: d

    The patient has the Currarino triad - most commonly associated with MNX1 mutation.

15. What is the mitotic activity that defines an atypical choroid plexus papilloma (WHO grade 2)?

    (a) >2 per 10 high power fields (HPFs)
    (b) >5 per 10 HPFs
    (c) >7 per 10 HPFs
    (d) >10 per 10 HPFs

    Answer: a

WHO classification of glioneuronal and neuronal tumors

- Ganglioglioma
- Desmoplastic infantile ganglioglioma/desmoplastic infantile astrocytoma
- Dysembryoplastic neuroepithelial tumor
- Diffuse glioneuronal tumor with oligodendroglioma-like features and nuclear clusters
- Papillary glioneuronal tumor
- Rosette-forming glioneuronal tumor
- Myxoid glioneuronal tumor
- Diffuse leptomeningeal glioneuronal tumor
- Gangliocytoma
- Multinodular and vacuolating neuronal tumor
- Dysplastic cerebellar gangliocytoma (Lhermitte-Duclos disease)
- Central neurocytoma
- Extraventricular neurocytoma
- Cerebellar liponeurocytoma

WHO classification of choroid plexus tumors

- Choroid plexus papilloma
- Atypical choroid plexus papilloma
- Choroid plexus carcinoma

Test your learning and check your understanding of this book's contents: use the "Springer Nature Flashcards" app to access questions using https://sn.pub/3HwHCw To use the app, please follow the instructions in Chap. 1.

Bibliography

1. Brzegowy K, Zarzecki MP, Musiał A, Aziz HM, Kasprzycki T, Tubbs RS, Popiela T, Walocha JA. The internal cerebral vein: new classification of branching patterns based on CTA. AJNR Am J Neuroradiol. 2019;40(10):1719–24. https://doi.org/10.3174/ajnr.A6200.
2. Altafulla JJ, Suh S, Bordes S, Prickett J, Iwanaga J, Loukas M, Dumont AS, Tubbs RS. Choroidal fissure and choroidal fissure cysts: a comprehensive review. Anat Cell Biol. 2020;53(2):121–5. https://doi.org/10.5115/acb.20.040.
3. Zohdi A, Elkheshin S. Endoscopic anatomy of the velum interpositum: a sequential descriptive anatomical study. Asian J Neurosurg. 2012;7(1):12–6. https://doi.org/10.4103/1793-5482.95689.
4. Rupareliya C, Naqvi S, Hejazi S. Alexia without agraphia: a rare entity. Cureus. 2017;9(6):e1304. https://doi.org/10.7759/cureus.1304.
5. Zhao X, Borba Moreira L, Cavallo C, Belykh E, Gandhi S, Labib MA, Tayebi Meybodi A, Mulholland CB, Liebelt BD, Lee M, Nakaji P, Preul MC. Quantitative endoscopic comparison of contralateral interhemispheric Transprecuneus and Supracerebellar Transtentorial Transcollateral sulcus approaches to the atrium. World Neurosurg. 2019;122:e215–25. https://doi.org/10.1016/j.wneu.2018.09.214.

6. Lee SJ, Bui TT, Chen CH, Lagman C, Chung LK, Sidhu S, Seo DJ, Yong WH, Siegal TL, Kim M, Yang I. Central neurocytoma: a review of clinical management and histopathologic features. Brain Tumor Res Treat. 2016;4(2):49–57. https://doi.org/10.14791/btrt.2016.4.2.49. Epub 2016 Oct 31

7. Park SJ, Jung TY, Kim SK, Lee KH. Tumor control of third ventricular central neurocytoma after gamma knife radiosurgery in an elderly patient: a case report and literature review. Medicine (Baltimore). 2018;97(50):e13657. https://doi.org/10.1097/MD.0000000000013657.

8. Safaee M, Oh MC, Bloch O, et al. Choroid plexus papillomas: advances in molecular biology and understanding of tumorigenesis. Neuro-Oncology. 2013;15(3):255–67. https://doi.org/10.1093/neuonc/nos289.

9. Beaumont TL, Limbrick DD Jr, Rich KM, Wippold FJ 2nd, Dacey RG Jr. Natural history of colloid cysts of the third ventricle. J Neurosurg. 2016;125(6):1420–30. https://doi.org/10.3171/2015.11.JNS151396. Epub 2016 Mar 11

10. Ravindran K, Sim K, Gaillard F. Magnetic resonance characterization of the 'dot sign' in colloid cysts of the third ventricle. J Clin Neurosci. 2019;62:133–7. https://doi.org/10.1016/j.jocn.2018.11.042. Epub 2018 Nov 27

11. Luo W, Xu Y, Yang J, Liu Z, Liu H. Fourth ventricular Meningiomas. World Neurosurg. 2019;127:e1201–9. https://doi.org/10.1016/j.wneu.2019.04.097. Epub 2019 Apr 17

12. Baalaan KP, Gurunathan N. Currarino triad. Pan Afr Med J. 2022;41:143. https://doi.org/10.11604/pamj.2022.41.143.33419.

Chapter 22
Miscellaneous Skull Base Tumors

Joe M Das

1. What is the most common sign of a skull base chordoma or chondrosarcoma?

   (a) Oculomotor nerve involvement
   (b) Abducens nerve involvement
   (c) Trigeminal motor involvement
   (d) Trigeminal sensory involvement

   Answer: b

2. Match the following paragangliomas with their sites of origin.

(a) Carotid body tumors	Auricular branch of the vagus
(b) Glomus jugulare tumors	Carotid bifurcation
(c) Glomus tympanicum tumors	Inferior vagal ganglion
(d) Glomus vagale tumors	Superior vagal ganglion

   Answer:

(a) Carotid body tumors	Carotid bifurcation
(b) Glomus jugulare tumors	Superior vagal ganglion
(c) Glomus tympanicum tumors	Auricular branch of the vagus
(d) Glomus vagale tumors	Inferior vagal ganglion

3. Weinstein-Boriani-Biagini classification system is used for

   (a) Pituitary tumors
   (b) Paragangliomas
   (c) Skull base meningiomas
   (d) Spinal tumors

   Answer: d

J. M. Das (✉)
Consultant Neurosurgeon, Bahrain Specialist Hospital, Juffair, Bahrain
e-mail: neurosurgeon@doctors.org.uk

© The Author(s), under exclusive license to Springer Nature
Switzerland AG 2023
J. M. Das, *Neuro-Oncology Explained Through Multiple Choice Questions*,
https://doi.org/10.1007/978-3-031-13253-7_22

- Fisch and Mattox classification—Jugular Paragangliomas
- Jackson-Glasscock classification—Jugulotympanic Paragangliomas
- Netterville-Glasscock classification—Vagal paragangliomas
- Shamblin classification—Carotid body tumors

4. Physaliphorous cells are characteristic of

   (a) Chordoma
   (b) Chondrosarcoma
   (c) Paraganglioma
   (d) Choroid plexus papilloma

   Answer: a

5. Which is the characteristic marker to identify a chordoma at biopsy?

   (a) Brachyury/T
   (b) S-100
   (c) K18
   (d) K19

   Answer: a

   Brachyury—a T-box transcription factor (6q27) that is essential for noto-chordal development.

6. Which is not a differentiating feature of ecchordosis physaliphora from chor-doma on radiological imaging?

   (a) Ecchordosis physaliphora are usually found to invade adjacent segments and the surrounding soft tissues
   (b) Ecchordosis physaliphora is osteosclerotic on computed tomogram scans
   (c) Ecchordosis physaliphora lacks significant contrast enhancement on MR images
   (d) Ecchordosis physaliphora has a negative uptake on technetium 99 m (^{99m}Tc) methylene diphosphonate bone scans

   Answer: a

   Notochordal rests- also known as benign notochordal cell tumors (BNCTs) or ecchordosis physaliphora (if located in the clivus).
   Ring-and-arc mineralization demonstrated with CT—chondrosarcoma

7. The usual line of treatment of chordomas and chondrosarcomas involves

   (a) En bloc R0 resection followed by high-dose radiotherapy
   (b) En bloc R0 resection
   (c) Neo-adjuvant radiotherapy followed by en bloc R0 resection
   (d) En bloc R0 resection followed by chemotherapy

   Answer: a

8. What is the most common type of succinate dehydrogenase mutation seen in hereditary head and neck paraganglioma?

(a) SDHA
(b) SDHB
(c) SDHC
(d) SDHD

Answer: d

- The highest prevalence and penetrance of all the SDH subunit mutations—*SDHD* mutation
- The highest risk of developing head and neck tumors is seen in relation to-*SDHD* (PGL1) and *SDHAF2* (PGL2).
- The highest risk for multiple PGLs—Mutations in *SDHD*
- The most commonly mutated gene in pheochromocytomas and extra-adrenal abdominal paragangliomas—*SDHB*
- The highest rate of metastasis in head and neck paragangliomas—Carriers of *SDHB* variants
- The highest risk for multifocal HNPGLs—Carriers of *SDHD/SDHAF2* mutations

9. Fontaine sign is clinically seen in

(a) Carotid paraganglioma
(b) Tympanic paraganglioma
(c) Jugular paraganglioma
(d) Vagal paraganglioma

Answer: a

- Carotid paraganglioma can usually be moved laterally, but not up or down due to its confinement within the carotid sheath—Fontaine sign
- Rising sun sign—Tympanic Paragangliomas
- Moth-eaten appearance of temporal bone— Jugular Paragangliomas
- The most aggressive paragangliomas and having the highest rate of metastasis—vagal paraganglioma

10. Which is the most sensitive tool for diagnosing head and neck paraganglioma?

(a) ^{18}F-FDOPA PET
(b) ^{68}Ga-DOTA-SST PET
(c) ^{18}F-FDG PET
(d) ^{111}In–labeled pentetreotide scintigraphy

Answer: b

Gallium 68–labeled dodecane tetraacetic acid-somatostatin analog (^{68}Ga-DOTA-SSTa) PET-CT

- Detects very small tumors, which can be missed by ^{18}F-FDOPA PET-CT
- The most sensitive tool for the detection of HNPs.

11. Preoperative embolization is not indicated in

(a) Carotid paraganglioma
(b) Tympanic paraganglioma
(c) Jugular paraganglioma
(d) Vagal paraganglioma

Answer: b

- First-line surgery—TPs and for CPs of Shamblin class I < 5 cm especially in young and relatively healthy patients.
- Surgery contraindicated in—bilateral synchronous CPs, due to the risk of baroreflex failure.
- Preoperative embolization to be considered in—JPs, CPs, and VPs
- No indication for preoperative embolization in TPs and LPs.
- First-line RT—large and growing JPs and VPs and large CPs.

12. Hyams grading system is used for

(a) Squamous cell carcinoma of paranasal sinuses
(b) Adenocarcinoma of paranasal sinuses
(c) Esthesioneuroblastoma
(d) Trigeminal schwannoma

Answer: c

Kadish and UCLA Staging Systems for-Esthesioneuroblastoma
Clavien–Dindo classification is a broadly accepted surgical complications classification system.

13. The Radkowski modification of the Sessions staging system is used for

(a) Squamous cell carcinoma of paranasal sinuses
(b) Juvenile nasopharyngeal angiofibroma
(c) Esthesioneuroblastoma
(d) Trigeminal schwannoma

Answer: b

Other staging systems—Chandler, Fisch, Önerci.

WHO Classification of Chondro-osseous Tumors

- Chondrogenic tumors
  - Mesenchymal chondrosarcoma
  - Chondrosarcoma
- Notochordal tumors
  - Chordoma (including poorly differentiated chordoma)

Test your learning and check your understanding of this book's contents: use the "Springer Nature Flashcards" app to access questions using https://sn.pub/3HwHCw To use the app, please follow the instructions in Chap. 1.

Bibliography

1. Volpe NJ, Liebsch NJ, Munzenrider JE, Lessell S. Neuro-ophthalmologic findings in chordoma and chondrosarcoma of the skull base. Am J Ophthalmol. 1993;115(1):97–104. https://doi.org/10.1016/s0002-9394(14)73531-7.
2. Pandiar D, Thammaiah S. Physaliphorous cells. J Oral Maxillofac Pathol. 2018;22(3):296–7. https://doi.org/10.4103/jomfp.JOMFP_265_18.
3. Jo VY, Hornick JL, Qian X. Utility of brachyury in distinction of chordoma from cytomorphologic mimics in fine-needle aspiration and core needle biopsy. Diagn Cytopathol. 2014;42(8):647–52. https://doi.org/10.1002/dc.23100. Epub 2014 Feb 19
4. Guha A, Vicha A, Zelinka T, Musil Z, Chovanec M. Genetic variants in patients with multiple head and neck Paragangliomas: dilemma in management. Biomedicine. 2021;9(6):626. Published 2021 May 31. https://doi.org/10.3390/biomedicines9060626.
5. Withey SJ, Perrio S, Christodoulou D, Izatt L, Carroll P, Velusamy A, Obholzer R, Lewington V, Jacques AET. Imaging features of succinate dehydrogenase-deficient Pheochromocytoma-Paraganglioma syndromes. Radiographics. 2019;39(5):1393–410. https://doi.org/10.1148/rg.2019180151.
6. Lin EP, Chin BB, Fishbein L, Moritani T, Montoya SP, Ellika S, Newlands S. Head and neck Paragangliomas: an update on the molecular classification, state-of-the-art imaging, and management recommendations. Radiol Imaging Cancer. 2022;4(3):e210088. https://doi.org/10.1148/rycan.210088.
7. Vuong HG, Ngo TNM, Dunn IF. Consolidating the Hyams grading system in esthesioneuroblastoma - an individual participant data meta-analysis. J Neuro-Oncol. 2021;153(1):15–22. https://doi.org/10.1007/s11060-021-03746-2. Epub 2021 Mar 26

Chapter 23
Primary CNS Lymphoma

Joe M Das

1. What is the most common type of primary CNS lymphoma?

   (a) Diffuse large B cell lymphoma
   (b) Burkitt lymphoma
   (c) T-lymphoblastic lymphoma
   (d) Follicular lymphoma

   Answer: a

2. Which of the following is the approximate 5-year survival rate for PCNSL?

   (a) 25%
   (b) 35%
   (c) 45%
   (d) 55%

   Answer: b

   The 5- and 10-year relative survival rates for PCNSL are 35.2% and 27.5%, respectively.

3. Which of the following is the only established risk factor for PCNSL?

   (a) Childhood exposure to radiation
   (b) Immunodeficiency
   (c) Infection with Ebstein-Barr Virus
   (d) Infection with JC virus

   Answer: b

J. M. Das (✉)
Consultant Neurosurgeon, Bahrain Specialist Hospital, Juffair, Bahrain
e-mail: neurosurgeon@doctors.org.uk

© The Author(s), under exclusive license to Springer Nature
Switzerland AG 2023
J. M. Das, *Neuro-Oncology Explained Through Multiple Choice Questions*,
https://doi.org/10.1007/978-3-031-13253-7_23

4. Which of the following is not a pan-B-cell marker?

   (a) CD2
   (b) CD19
   (c) CD20
   (d) CD79a

   Answer: a

   - Most tumors express pan– B-cell markers, including CD19, CD20, CD22, and CD79a.
   - T-cell markers include CD2 and CD3.

5. Which subtype of PCNSL has the worst prognosis?

   (a) Type 2 large B-cell lymphoma
   (b) Type 3 large B-cell lymphoma
   (c) Germinal center B-cell-like lymphoma (GCB)
   (d) Activated B-cell–like (ABC) lymphoma

   Answer: d

   Three molecular subclasses are defined by gene expression profiling

   - Type 3 large B-cell lymphoma
   - Germinal center B-cell-like lymphoma (GCB)
   - Activated B-cell–like (ABC) lymphoma

   PCNSL has a high prevalence of the ABC gene expression profile sub-type → relatively inferior prognosis of this lymphoma.

6. Which of the following mutations is found commonly in PCNSL?

   (a) *TOX*
   (b) *CARD11*
   (c) *TNFAIP3*
   (d) *MYD88*

   Answer: d

   Pathogenesis of PCNSL is by two mechanisms:

   - MYD88 and CD79B mutations lead to Toll-like receptor (TLR) signaling.
   - Concurrent B-cell receptor pathway activation

   The most common mutation of MYD88 is missense mutation at L265P.

7. Which of the following is an unlikely MRI brain finding in PCNSL?

   (a) Restricted diffusion leading to a hyperintense signal b-1000
   (b) Hypointense signal on ADC images
   (c) Large choline peak
   (d) Large NAA peak

   Answer: d

8. Which of the following is not a poor prognostic factor for PCNSL?

   (a) Elevated serum level of lactate dehydrogenase
   (b) Elevated CSF protein
   (c) Involvement of non-hemispheric areas of the brain
   (d) Age < 60 years

   Answer: d

9. Which is the most effective chemotherapeutic agent for the treatment of PCNSL?

   (a) Methotrexate
   (b) Vincristine
   (c) Paclitaxel
   (d) Carboplatin

   Answer: a

   - The most effective treatment for PCNSL is intravenous, high-dose methotrexate (>3 g/m^2). The induction treatment should include Rituximab as well.

10. Early intervention with which of the following drugs can reduce nephrotoxicity due to high dose methotrexate?

    (a) Thioredocin
    (b) Polyhistidine
    (c) Glutathione S-transferase
    (d) Glucarpidase

    Answer: d

    - Glucarpidase is a recombinant form of carboxypeptidase-G2 produced from *Escherichia coli*.

11. Ibrutinib, used in the treatment of PCNSL, works by which of the following mechanisms?

    (a) PI3K inhibitor
    (b) BTK inhibitor
    (c) mTOR inhibitor
    (d) Dual PI3K/mTOR inhibitor

    Answer: b

    - Temsorolimus is an mTOR inhibitor.
    - Buparlisib is a pan-PI3K inhibitor.

12. Which of the following is a novel prognostic marker for PCNSL?

    (a) Neutrophil-to-lymphocyte ratio
    (b) Derived neutrophil-to-lymphocyte ratio
    (c) Lactate dehydrogenase-to-lymphocyte ratio
    (d) Glutathione reductase-to-lymphocyte ratio

    Answer: c

13. Which of the following is not a component in the International Extranodal Lymphoma Study Group (IELSG) prognostic score?

    (a) Age
    (b) CSF protein concentration
    (c) Deep brain involvement
    (d) Sex

    Answer: d

    The components of the IELSG Score are:
    • Age
    • Eastern Cooperative Oncology Group performance score
    • Lactate dehydrogenase level
    • CSF protein concentration and
    • Deep brain involvement (periventricular regions, basal ganglia, brainstem, and/or cerebellum)

    2-year survival rate

    • 0–1 risk factors—80%
    • 2–3—48%
    • 4–5—15%

14. Which of the following drugs is not a part of the MATRix regimen that has been shown to be associated with better survival in primary CNS lymphoma?

    (a) Methotrexate
    (b) Cytarabine
    (c) Cyclophosphamide
    (d) Thiotepa

    Answer: c

15. The most frequent genomic aberrations in primary CNS lymphoma involve the losses and deletions involving which chromosome?

    (a) 6p21
    (b) 22p21
    (c) 6q21
    (d) 22q21

    Answer: a

16. Match the following novel agents being tried in the treatment of primary CNS lymphoma with their mechanisms of action:

(a) Lenalidomide	Inhibition of PI3K
(b) Ibrutinib	Small molecule inhibitor of mTOR
(c) Temsirolimus	Modulation of the substrate specificity of the CRL4^{CRBN} E3 ubiquitin ligase
(d) Buparlisib	Bruton's tyrosine kinase inhibitor

Answer:

(a) Lenalidomide	Modulation of the substrate specificity of the CRL4^{CRBN} E3 ubiquitin ligase
(b) Ibrutinib	Bruton's tyrosine kinase inhibitor
(c) Temsirolimus	Small molecule inhibitor of mTOR
(d) Buparlisib	Inhibition of PI3K

17. A 40-year-old immunocompetent patient comes to the outpatient department with complains of mild headaches and left-sided weakness for the past week. Clinically, he is conscious and oriented. Pronator drift is positive on the left side. There is no papilledema. An MRI scan of the brain shows a T1 and T2 hypointense lesion in the right basal ganglia region measuring 2 × 1 cm which shows a reduced ADC and mild perilesional edema. It is enhancing strongly on contrast administration. Given the suspicion of CNS lymphoma, what is the next step in the management of this patient?

(a) Whole body contrast-CT scan
(b) Stereotactic biopsy
(c) Ophthalmological evaluation
(d) CSF examination

Answer: a

- The initial line of investigation involves physical examination, routine blood studies, contrast CT scan of the whole body, [18]FDG PET, and an ultrasound scan of the testes.

WHO classification of hematolymphoid tumors of the CNS

Lymphomas
- CNS lymphomas
  - Primary diffuse large B-cell lymphoma of the CNS
  - Immunodeficiency-associated CNS lymphoma
  - Lymphomatoid granulomatosis
  - Intravascular large B-cell lymphoma
- Miscellaneous rare lymphomas in the CNS
  - MALT lymphoma of the dura
  - Other low-grade B-cell lymphomas of the CNS
  - Anaplastic large cell lymphoma (ALK+/ALK−)
  - T-cell and NK/T-cell lymphomas

Histiocytic tumors
- Erdheim-Chester disease
- Rosai-Dorfman disease
- Juvenile xanthogranuloma
- Langerhans cell histiocytosis
- Histiocytic sarcoma

Test your learning and check your understanding of this book's contents: use the "Springer Nature Flashcards" app to access questions using https://sn.pub/3HwHCw To use the app, please follow the instructions in Chap. 1.

Bibliography

1. Grommes C, DeAngelis LM. Primary CNS lymphoma. J Clin Oncol. 2017;35(21):2410–8. https://doi.org/10.1200/JCO.2017.72.7602. Epub 2017 Jun 22
2. Ostrom QT, Cioffi G, Gittleman H, Patil N, Waite K, Kruchko C, Barnholtz-Sloan JS. CBTRUS statistical report: primary brain and other central nervous system tumors diagnosed in the United States in 2012–2016. Neuro-Oncology. 2019;21(Suppl 5):v1–v100. https://doi.org/10.1093/neuonc/noz150.
3. Gerstner ER, Batchelor TT. Primary central nervous system lymphoma. Arch Neurol. 2010;67(3):291–7. https://doi.org/10.1001/archneurol.2010.3.
4. Kumar V, Shrivastava SM, TrishalaMeghal T, Chandra BA. Recent advances in diffuse large B cell lymphoma. In: Guenova M, Balatzenko G, editors. Hematology - latest research and clinical advances [Internet]. London: IntechOpen; 2018. [cited 2022 Jun 15]. https://www.intechopen.com/chapters/60573. https://doi.org/10.5772/intechopen.74263.
5. Chen K, Ma Y, Ding T, Zhang X, Chen B, Guan M. Effectiveness of digital PCR for MYD88^{L265P} detection in vitreous fluid for primary central nervous system lymphoma diagnosis. Exp Ther Med. 2020;20(1):301–8. https://doi.org/10.3892/etm.2020.8695. Epub 2020 Apr 29
6. Lukas RV, Stupp R, Gondi V, et al. Primary central nervous system lymphoma-PART 1: Epidemiology, diagnosis, staging, and prognosis. Oncology (Williston Park). 2018;32(1):17–22.
7. Schaff LR, Lobbous M, Carlow D, Schofield R, Gavrilovic IT, Miller AM, Stone JB, Piotrowski AF, Sener U, Skakodub A, Acosta EP, Ryan KJ, Mellinghoff IK, DeAngelis LM, Nabors LB, Grommes C. Routine use of low-dose glucarpidase following high-dose methotrexate in adult patients with CNS lymphoma: an open-label, multi-center phase I study. BMC Cancer. 2022;22(1):60. https://doi.org/10.1186/s12885-021-09164-x.
8. Robak E, Robak T. Bruton's kinase inhibitors for the treatment of immunological diseases: current status and perspectives. J Clin Med. 2022;11(10):2807. https://doi.org/10.3390/jcm11102807.
9. Gao Y, Wei L, Kim SJ, Wang L, He Y, Zheng Y, Bertero L, Pellerino A, Cassoni P, Tamagnone L, Theresa PK, Deutsch A, Zhan H, Lai J, Wang Y, You H. A novel prognostic marker for primary CNS lymphoma: lactate dehydrogenase-to-lymphocyte ratio improves stratification of patients within the low and intermediate MSKCC risk groups. Front Oncol. 2021;3(11):696147. https://doi.org/10.3389/fonc.2021.696147.
10. Ferreri AJM. Therapy of primary CNS lymphoma: role of intensity, radiation, and novel agents. Hematology Am Soc Hematol Educ Program. 2017;2017(1):565–77. https://doi.org/10.1182/asheducation-2017.1.565.
11. Fink EC, Ebert BL. The novel mechanism of lenalidomide activity. Blood. 2015;126(21):2366–9. https://doi.org/10.1182/blood-2015-07-567958. Epub 2015 Oct 5

Chapter 24
Palliative Care

Amr Maani, Abduelmenem Alashkham, and Jacek Baj

1. A 61-year-old male patient presents to the clinic with a history of headaches and current personality changes. An MRI of the brain has confirmed a diagnosis of Grade 4 astrocytoma. What is the approximate survival rate for a patient with glioblastoma?

   (a) 3–5 years
   (b) 1–1.5 years
   (c) 12–15 years
   (d) 1–2 months
   (e) None of the above

   Answer: b

   A patient with grade 4 astrocytoma has approximately a survival time between 12 and 18 months. On the other hand, the approximate survival time for grade 2 is 5–10 years and for grade 3 it is 2–3 years. The prognosis can be altered by certain factors such as age, neurologic deficits, treatment options, etc. Treatment options can play a role in survival. For example, the use of temozolomide alongside radiotherapy showed a higher median survival rate compared to the use of radiotherapy alone.

2. A 62-year-old female is diagnosed with an incurable brain tumor. End-of-life (EoL) treatment decisions are provided for the alleviation of the symptoms in

A. Maani (✉)
Department of Anatomy, Medical University of Lublin, Lublin, Poland
e-mail: 2439022@dundee.ac.uk

A. Alashkham
Edinburgh Medical School, The University of Edinburgh, Edinburgh, UK

J. Baj
Chair and Department of Anatomy, Medical University of Lublin, Lublin, Poland

© The Author(s), under exclusive license to Springer Nature Switzerland AG 2023
J. M. Das, *Neuro-Oncology Explained Through Multiple Choice Questions*,
https://doi.org/10.1007/978-3-031-13253-7_24

incurable brain tumor patients. They include withholding, withdrawing, and terminal sedation. Which of the following option best describes withdrawing?

(a) Not to accept symptomatic therapies which were otherwise warranted in a planned decision
(b) Symptomatic treatment withdrawal that has been ongoing
(c) Complete loss of consciousness by the pharmacologically induced reduction of vigilance up to abolish or reduce the perception of symptoms that could be intolerable
(d) Options a and b are correct
(e) None of the above

Answer: b

Not accepting symptomatic therapies which were otherwise warranted in a planned decision describes withholding. Symptomatic treatment withdrawal that has been ongoing correctly describes withdrawing. Lastly, a complete loss of consciousness by the pharmacologically induced reduction of vigilance up describes terminal sedation.

3. A 64-year-old male patient presented to the clinic with complaints of frequent episodes of epilepsy. He has been recently diagnosed with high-grade glioma and is currently undergoing chemotherapy sessions. As interactions of AEDs, steroids, and chemotherapy are common, which is the preferred drug of choice that will help in the management of this patient?

(a) Gabapentin
(b) Levetiracetam
(c) Valproic acid
(d) Options a and b
(e) Bevacizumab

Answer: d

Gabapentin is an anticonvulsant recommended for treating epilepsy in patients undergoing chemotherapy. Levetiracetam is also a drug of choice in patients with epilepsy who are undergoing chemotherapy sessions. Valproic acid is normally the first-choice agent. However, it may increase the toxicity of chemotherapy as an enzyme inhibitor. Thus, both drugs are considered to be the best-tolerated drugs as well as the most effective. Bevacizumab is not applicable for treating epilepsy as well as not recommended in managing VTE in malignant glioma patients because it may further increase the risk of VTE.

4. A 83-year-old female patient undergoing whole brain radiotherapy for the past 6 months for a high-grade brain tumor presented with complaints of memory disturbances, and a deterioration of complex intellectual functions with mood and personality changes. The patient also complains of slowed thinking and processing of information. Complaints of aphasias, apraxias, and agnosias are absent. Frontal sub-cortical dementia is suspected. What would be the drug of choice for this patient?

(a) Methylprednisolone
(b) Methylphenidate
(c) Valproic acid
(d) Rivastigmine
(e) None of the above

Answer: b

Methylprednisolone is a corticosteroid that is used for anti-inflammatory purposes. Methylphenidate is proven effective in dealing with irreversible frontal subcortical dementia in elderly patients undergoing whole-brain radiotherapy or chemotherapy. Valproic acid is an anticonvulsant used to treat seizures. Rivastigmine is a cholinesterase inhibitor used for the treatment of mild to moderate degenerative brain disorders causing memory and thinking problems. However, it is not effective in irreversible subcortical dementia.

5. A 64-year-old male patient being treated for an end-stage glioma is complaining of myalgias and arthralgias. He has been taking steroids for the past 12 months, which could result in myopathy and osteoporosis. Which would be the best course of action in dealing with patients if steroids are a necessary part of treatment in advanced stages?

(a) Provide adequate nutritional support to the patient (calcium, protein, vitamin D)
(b) Suggest an adequate daily physical activity
(c) Recommend physiotherapy sessions
(d) If needed, a slow tapering of steroids is recommended
(e) All of the above

Answer: e

Option A is correct as adequate nutrition helps in decreasing the rate of osteoporosis as well as increasing muscle strength. Physical activity is necessary to load the weakened muscles and increase their strength. A diffuse myalgia/arthralgia withdrawal syndrome is usually caused by a fast tapering of steroids. A slower tapering of steroids is recommended. Thus, all of the options combined are the best course of action in dealing with this issue.

6. A 32-year-old male is diagnosed with end-stage brain cancer. He has been experiencing fatigue daily. What is the best course of action that will help brain cancer patients with their fatigue?

(a) Light daily exercise
(b) Methylphenidate
(c) Ginseng
(d) Erythropoietin and darbepoetin-alpha
(e) Options a and d

Answer: e

Fatigue in end-stage brain cancer is a very common symptom. Daily exercise in a tolerance zone is recommended in brain cancer patients to counter fatigue symptoms as well as to preserve conditioning. Currently, a combination therapy with ginseng and methylphenidate is under review for dealing with fatigue in brain cancer patients regarding its efficacy and safety. Darbopoietin alpha and erythropoietin are considered to be common treatment options for chemotherapy-related anemia that causes fatigue. Weekly, as well as bimonthly administration, helps in the patient's day-to-day life.

7. A 61-year-old male patient is undergoing treatment for low-grade glioma. The patient has presented to the clinic with complaints of changes in appetite and weight loss. Which of the following treatments can help in increasing the appetite of this patient?

(a) Steroids
(b) Valproic acid
(c) Topiramate
(d) Options a and b
(e) None of the above

Answer: d

Steroids are indicated in brain tumor patients, especially in end-stage treatment. They are known to increase the appetite of the patient. Just like steroids, valproic acid also increases the appetite of the patient. Thus, both options A and B are correct in this case. Topiramate has the opposite effect in which it decreases the appetite in patients.

8. A 34-year-old female patient diagnosed with high-grade glioma presented to the emergency department with frequent episodes of seizures. The prognosis of this patient is poor and she is currently being treated at home. What should the preferred mode of AEDs administration be for this patient?

(a) Oral
(b) Intravenous
(c) Intramuscular
(d) Oral and intravenous
(e) None of the above

Answer: c

The oral route for AEDs can be problematic for patients having end-stage brain tumors owing to swallowing difficulties, mostly those caused by alterations of consciousness as well as dysphagia. The intravenous route is preferred in medical facilities for fast response. Thus, intramuscular along with transdermal, rectal, and subcutaneous routes are preferred in home settings.

9. A 56-year-old male patient is diagnosed with glioblastoma multiforme. Even after aggressive and multidisciplinary treatment with chemotherapy, radiotherapy, and surgery, the prognosis for both primary as well as metastatic brain

tumors continues to be poor. What is the median survival rate for glioblastoma multiforme?

(a) 7 to 8 years
(b) 12 to 15 months
(c) 2 to 5 years
(d) 3 to 4 years
(e) None of the above

Answer: b

Typically, the prognosis for metastatic brain and the primary tumors is poor. Malignant gliomas are considered to have the poorest outcome. Thus, 12 to 15 months is the median survival rate for glioblastoma multiforme. On the other hand, 2 to 5 years is the survival rate for anaplastic gliomas. The rest of the options are incorrect.

10. A 73-year-old female patient, known to have a glioma presented to the clinic with complaints of headache and dizziness. The patient also suffered from frequent episodes of vomiting and neck stiffness. On MRI, peritumoral brain edema has been confirmed. The physician is planning to prescribe either dexamethasone or methylprednisolone for the chronic treatment of peritumoral brain edema. What should the recommended dosage of dexamethasone and methylprednisolone respectively be?

(a) 96 mg and 8 mg given once or twice daily
(b) 8 mg and 96 mg are given once or twice daily
(c) 96 and 8 mg given thrice daily
(d) 8 mg and 96 mg given thrice daily
(e) 8 mg and 96 mg are given only once daily

Answer: b

A corticosteroid such as dexamethasone is considered to be an effective drug in reducing tissue edema by reducing vascular permeability. It has a longer half-life, which allows patients to take it once a day. Methylprednisolone is a corticosteroid that is used for anti-inflammatory purposes. Thus, option B is the recommended dosage respectively.

11. A 60-year-old female patient who is diagnosed with malignant glioma. It has been shown in previous studies that malignant glioma patients are usually at a high risk of developing venous thromboembolism (VTE). Certain drugs are used to help in both the treatment of symptomatic VTE as well as the prevention of recurrent VTE among cancer patients but not in malignant glioma patients. What are those drugs?

(a) Bevacizumab
(b) Low molecular weight heparin (LMWH)
(c) Erythropoietin
(d) Darbopoietin-alpha
(e) Bevacizumab and LMWH

Answer: e

In spite of the fact that there is doubt about the efficacy of the use of primary prophylaxis among cancer patients, certain drugs such as bevacizumab and LMWH are used in both the treatment of symptomatic VTE and its prevention. However, bevacizumab is not recommended for managing VTE in malignant glioma patients because it may further increase the risk of VTE.

12. A 63-year-old male patient who is diagnosed with high-grade glioma presents with gradual shortness of breath and chest tightness. The patient's body temperature is also increased and there is audible wheezing. The patient is taking steroids for the past 6 months for his brain tumor. What could be the most probable diagnosis?

    (a) *Pneumocystis jirovecii* pneumonitis (PJP)
    (b) Acute respiratory distress syndrome (ARDS)
    (c) Lymphocytic interstitial pneumonia (LIP)
    (d) Chronic obstructive pulmonary disease (COPD)
    (e) None of the above

    Answer: a

    A clinically major suppression of the immune system is produced from common use of corticosteroids, which could lead to opportunistic infections to occur such as PJP. ARDS normally appears in patients who are in critical condition. The main symptom is severe shortness of breath (SOB) which occurs within a few hours or days after an infection or an injury. Since this patient developed SOB gradually, ARDS is not the correct option. LIP is associated with lymphoproliferative and autoimmune disorders, which include pernicious anemia, rheumatoid arthritis, myasthenia gravis, and Hashimoto thyroiditis. LIP is a syndrome of fever, dyspnea, and cough, along with bibasilar pulmonary infiltrates comprising dense interstitial buildups of plasma cells and lymphocytes. COPD causes airflow obstruction and breathing-associated complications, which includes chronic bronchitis and emphysema.

13. A 54-year-old male patient, a diagnosed case of glioma presented to you with complaints of frequent headaches. You suspect it to be due to vasogenic edema. What would be the first choice to treat this type of headache?

    (a) Dexamethasone
    (b) Opioids
    (c) Non-Steroidal Anti-Inflammatory Drugs (NSAIDs)
    (d) Anticonvulsants
    (e) Opioids along with anticonvulsants

    Answer: a

    Dexamethasone is the first choice of clinicians in managing headaches in glioma patients due to vasogenic edema. Options B and C are used for managing pain in glioma patients, but they are not the first choice. Option D is mainly used for seizure management.

14. A 63-year-old male patient presents with subacute onset of apraxia and new headaches. The headaches are present when the patient first awakens and, at times, they wake him from sleep. More recently, they have been associated with nausea and vomiting. An MRI scan shows the single nature of the lesion and the heterogeneous nonspherical enhancement pattern, which suggests a diagnosis of a high-grade primary brain tumor such as glioblastoma, the most common glioma in adults. Which of the following is associated with a greater survival in glioblastoma?

    (a) Bevacizumab added to up-front treatment with radiation therapy and temozolomide
    (b) Age greater than 65 years at diagnosis
    (c) MGMT promoter methylation presence
    (d) Neoadjuvant chemotherapy before radiation therapy
    (e) All except option c

    Answer: c

    Evidence does not support the use of up-front treatment with bevacizumab, an anti-vascular endothelial growth factor antibody, added to chemoradiation with temozolomide in the majority of patients with glioblastoma. Advanced age, in general, represents a significant survival disadvantage. O6-methylguanine-DNA-methyltransferase (MGMT) is a repair enzyme that removes excessive methyl groups from DNA, mitigating the effects of DNA damage induced by chemotherapy agents and radiation therapy. Silencing of the MGMT gene via methylation of its promoter is a favorable prognostic biomarker. It also predicts prolonged survival with the use of temozolomide for glioblastoma. Neoadjuvant chemotherapy has been investigated in newly diagnosed glioblastoma. At this time, there is no evidence to support the use of chemotherapy before radiation therapy in this tumor type.

15. A 70-year-old male patient with complaints of headache, nausea, vomiting, vision disorders (double vision), and deteriorating consciousness. The patient is a known case of glioma and is currently on chemotherapy and radiotherapy. Dexamethasone is considered the standard choice for dealing with vasogenic brain edema. Which of the following is the main reason behind choosing this corticosteroid to treat vasogenic brain edema?

    (a) Longer half-life
    (b) The absence of mineralocorticoid effect
    (c) Low inhibition of leucocyte migration
    (d) Options b and c
    (e) All of the above

    Answer: e

    Dexamethasone has a longer half-life as compared to the other corticosteroids. Dexamethasone does not have any mineralocorticoid effect. There is low inhibition of leucocytic migration when dexamethasone is used. Thus, the entire characteristics mentioned in the rest of the answers make dexamethasone the drug of choice.

16. Glioma patients are at a greater risk of acquiring Deep Vein Thrombosis (DVT). Tumor surgery could also lead to a hypercoagulable state, in which a release of thrombotic microparticles could occur. Neurosurgical data recommends a "triple" prophylaxis to DVT in glioma patients, which consists of?

    (a) Limb setting, pneumatic compression, and Low Molecular Weight Heparin (LMWH)
    (b) Preventive aspirin and Low Molecular Weight Heparin (LMWH)
    (c) Pneumatic compression and limb setting
    (d) Low Molecular Weight Heparin (LMWH)
    (e) Limb setting and preventive aspirin

    Answer: a

    Neurosurgical data recommends a "triple" prophylaxis to Deep Vein Thrombosis (DVT), which includes limb setting, pneumatic compression, and Low Molecular Weight Heparin (LMWH). However, aspirin is not recommended for the prevention of DVT in glioma patients.

17. A 72-year-old female patient presented to your clinic with complaints of headache. Based on your research, a prescription of dexamethasone is given to this patient. Which of the following can be an associated symptom of dexamethasone that becomes worse with the increase in the dosage or duration of the treatment in patients with glioma?

    (a) Cushing's effect
    (b) Diabetes mellitus
    (c) Muscle weakness
    (d) Malignant hyperthermia
    (e) All except option d

    Answer: e

    Cushing's effect, muscle weakness, and diabetes are the most common symptoms associated with the use of dexamethasone in patients with glioma. Nonetheless, dexamethasone is the preferred choice of drug to manage headaches in a patient with glioma. Malignant hyperthermia is not a side effect of dexamethasone. It is a side effect of succinylcholine, which is an anesthetic agent.

18. A 38-year-old male patient is being treated for a grade 4-brain tumor that has a very poor prognosis. Based on current evidence regarding the patient's condition, which of the following symptoms is most common at the end of life in such patients?

    (a) Swallowing disorders
    (b) Headaches
    (c) Insomnia
    (d) Epilepsy
    (e) Delirium

    Answer: a

Swallowing disorders are usually present in 85% of end-of-life cases. Headaches are present in 36% of the cases. Epilepsy is present in 30% of the cases. Insomnia is incorrect. Delirium is present in 15% of the cases. Thus, option A is correct.

19. A 54-year-old patient presented to the emergency room with complaints of episodes of seizures and motor weakness. The patient is drowsy and has difficulty speaking. The patient's caregiver reports personality changes in the patient for the past few months. You suspect a malignant brain tumor. Which of the following tumors is the largely common malignant central nervous system (CNS) tumor?

    (a) Grade 4; Low-grade gliomas
    (b) Grade 4; High-grade gliomas
    (c) Grade 4; Ependymoma
    (d) Grade 4; Meningioma
    (e) Options b and c

    Answer: b

    The largely common primary malignant central nervous system (CNS) tumor is Grade 4 high-grade gliomas according to the World Health Organization (WHO). Episodes of seizures, motor weakness, personality changes, drowsiness, and difficulty in speaking can occur in common primary CNS tumors. Thus, the rest of the options are incorrect.

20. A neuro-oncology physician is seeing multiple brain cancer patients in an oncology ward and the majority of them have seizure complaints. The physician is directed to choose a drug depending on each patient's comorbidities and other medications. After research, the physician finds out that levetiracetam is the most commonly used drug to treat seizures. Which of the following options makes this drug a favorable choice?

    (a) Less interaction with mood disorders
    (b) Less interaction with anxiety disorders
    (c) Metabolism through the liver
    (d) Ease of titration
    (e) Options c and d

    Answer: d

    Options A and B are not correct because the main common cause to discontinue levetiracetam is irritability. Thus, it is usually avoided in patients with anxiety or a mood disorder. Levetiracetam is a favorable choice due to its ease of titration, which results in a favorable side effect profile. Lastly, option C is incorrect, since it is metabolized through the kidney and not the liver.

21. Palliative care is an important aspect of dealing with patients suffering from incurable brain tumors with poor prognoses. Which of the following best describes the "patient and caregiver needs" aspect of palliative care?

(a) Multidisciplinary support programs that address the patient's problem, which help to reduce the burden on the patient and caregivers.
(b) Care strategies must be changed after every evaluation.
(c) Palliative care only deals with the medical needs of the patient
(d) Psychological support is not a part of palliative care
(e) Our main concern in palliative care is to prolong the life of the patient at any cost.

Answer: a

Palliative care via multidisciplinary programs is applied to address patients' needs and help to reduce their burden. Standards of care might also be enhanced proactively, thus extending care goals beyond medical needs. Continuous re-evaluation of the patient's support needs and the need for information is necessary because the patient's needs may change with the progression of the disease. Care strategies should be amended accordingly (It is not mandatory to change strategies after every evaluation). Palliative care is aimed to provide the best available support to the patient. This may also extend beyond just medical needs. Psychological support is also included in palliative care as it addresses the symptoms like depression, especially at the end-of-life stage.

22. A 63-year-old male patient is seen for grade 2 meningioma and he has been using high-dose corticosteroids (dexamethasone) for the past 6 months. Recently, the patient has been experiencing significant side effects which led to a worsening in his quality of life. Thus, the patient's physician decided to initiate a tapering plan. Which of the following options is an indicator that the physician can start tapering the dose of corticosteroids?

(a) The tumor is a response to the patient's systemic treatment
(b) Post-radiation edema is being resolved with time
(c) Surgical removal of the tumor previously
(d) The tumor has been surgically debulked
(e) All of the above

Answer: e

If high doses of corticosteroids are used for long durations, significant side effects can develop that can paradoxically lead to deterioration in the patient's quality of life. Thus, the dosage of corticosteroids should be tapered slowly if the tumor is responding to systemic treatment. If post-radiation is resolving with time, it is also an indication of initiating a tapering plan. There is no need for high-dose steroids if the tumor has been removed surgically.

23. A 55-year-old female patient was diagnosed with a primary brain tumor. While the prognosis of primary brain tumor patients continues to remain poor, a variety of treatment options are used. Cytotoxic chemotherapy is considered to be part of the care provided for the majority of glioma patients. Which of the following is a common side effect of chemotherapy with vincristine?

(a) Delayed wound healing
(b) Pulmonary fibrosis

(c) Neuropathy
(d) Skin rash
(e) Hypertension

Answer: c

Option A is incorrect, delayed wound healing is a main side effect of Bevacizumab. Option B is incorrect, pulmonary fibrosis is a side effect of Lomustine. Neuropathy is a common side effect of vincristine, thus, C is correct. Option D is incorrect; skin rash is a common side effect of temozolomide and procarbazine. Hypertension is considered to be a common side effect of bevacizumab.

24. A 67-year-old male patient who was diagnosed with grade 2 astrocytoma presented to emergency with a single episode of seizure. The patient is in fear of getting hospitalized and is restless. What should be the acute treatment of seizures used for brain tumor patients?

(a) Benzodiazepine
(b) Succinylcholine
(c) Phenytoin
(d) Benzodiazepine and phenytoin
(e) Succinylcholine and phenytoin

Answer: d

Benzodiazepine is usually used to terminate status epilepticus or a seizure. In addition, intravenous (IV) phenytoin is also used to prevent a recurrence. Succinylcholine is not considered to be an anesthetic agent.

25. A 43-year-old female patient, diagnosed case of glioblastoma has presented to the emergency department (ED) with complaints of body aches, gradual muscular weakness, and dry skin. The patient's blood pressure (BP) is 179/100 and respiratory rate (RR) is 24. On inquiring, the ED physician gets to know that the patient has been taking corticosteroids for the past 2 years. To avoid any further complications, the physician plans to switch this patient from corticosteroid to another alternative drug. Which drug is most likely to be recommended?

(a) Dexamethasone
(b) Valproic Acid
(c) Bevacizumab
(d) Options a and b
(e) All of the above

Answer: c

Dexamethasone is a steroid and cannot be used, as it will further aggravate the symptoms of this patient. Valproic acid is an anticonvulsant and is not suitable for this patient, as his primary complaints do not include seizures. Bevacizumab therapy is favored for its use in recurrent high-grade glioma. It can also be taken into consideration in an event when a patient is incapable to be weaned off or reduced to a low dose of corticosteroids. This monoclonal antibody binds to the vascular endothelial growth factor. Due to its angioedema characteristics, this drug could be a palliative medication that is beneficial for patients.

26. A 39-year-old female patient was diagnosed with a primary brain cancer tumor (glioma). Although the patient's prognosis remains generally poor, a variety of treatment options can be used as standard care such as cytotoxic chemotherapy. Which of the following is a common side effect of chemotherapy combined with temozolomide?

    (a) Reversible posterior leukoencephalopathy syndrome
    (b) Hypertension
    (c) *Pneumocystis jirovecii* pneumonia
    (d) Skin rash
    (e) Delayed wound healing

    Answer: c

    Reversible posterior leukoencephalopathy syndrome is a common side effect of bevacizumab as well as hypertension, thus, options A and B are incorrect. Option C is correct; *Pneumocystis jirovecii* pneumonia is a common side effect of temozolomide. Option D is incorrect since skin rash is a common side effect of temozolomide as well as procarbazine. Delayed wound healing is a main side effect of bevacizumab.

27. Which of the following is the main reason behind the disability in patients with end-stage brain tumors that also increases the risks of thromboembolic complications?

    (a) Epilepsy
    (b) Fatigue
    (c) Headache
    (d) Focal deficits
    (e) Stiffness syndrome

    Answer: d

    Epilepsy or seizures is a major symptom in patients with brain tumors, especially near the end-of-life stage but that does not increase the risk of thromboembolic complications. Fatigue is also the main complaint in patients with a brain tumor but is not related to the given scenario. Headache is the major complaint in brain tumors mostly because of the extra stress of the tumor mass or increased intracranial pressure, but that is not the reason behind the disability of the patient. However, focal deficits, mainly the motor ones, impair the quality of life and autonomy of the patient which exposes the patient to thromboembolic complications and eventually, leads to physical disability.

28. A 63-year-old male patient, diagnosed case of low-grade glioma, presented to the emergency department with complaints of cognitive issues. The patient is taking multiple medications for his tumor for the past 1-year. Which of the following might be the reason behind the intellectual impairment in this patient?

(a) Anti-epileptic drugs
(b) Corticosteroids
(c) NSAIDs
(d) Chemotherapy
(e) Radiotherapy

Answer: a

Recent studies found that in patients with low-grade glioma the use of anti-epileptic drugs is the main reason behind cognitive impairments. Corticosteroids are associated with complaints of weakness along with Cushing's effect and diabetes mellites. The use of NSAIDs is not associated with cognitive complications in people with brain tumors. Chemotherapy and radiotherapy are also associated with cognitive impairments in brain tumor patients, but AEDs are the most likely reason behind cognitive impairments in patients with low-grade glioma.

29. A 43-year-old female patient having grade 4 glioblastoma presented to the clinic due to worsening symptoms. The prognosis for this patient is poor. What should be the role of a multidisciplinary brain tumor program in palliative care?

(a) To deliver a tailored understanding of the diagnosis
(b) To provide needed knowledge about the prognosis
(c) To offer information regarding the treatment options
(d) To deliver tailored education regarding the recurrence as well as end-of-life care
(e) All of the above are correct

Answer: e

To prolong life is not the goal of palliative care at all. Quality of life should be maintained or improved throughout the progression of the disease as much as possible. Education about the prognosis is a part not the main role of the multidisciplinary brain tumor program. Treating just the symptoms is not the complete approach of a multidisciplinary program. Thus, providing knowledge regarding the diagnosis, treatment options, prognosis, recurrence, and end-of-life care helps in reducing the psychosocial effect in patients.

30. A corticosteroid such as dexamethasone is a commonly prescribed medication for patients who are diagnosed with a brain tumor. What is the mechanism of this analgesic agent?

(a) Decreases vascular permeability
(b) Offers low potency
(c) Inhibits the synthesis of prostaglandin
(d) Has a short half-life
(e) Options a and c

Answer: e

A corticosteroid such as dexamethasone is an effective drug in controlling the symptoms in patients with a brain tumor. This drug is known to cause less fluid retention and helps in reducing tissue edema by reducing vascular permeability. It has a longer half-life which allows patients to take it once daily. Lastly, it reduces inflammation as a result of inhibiting prostaglandin synthesis.

31. A 66-year-old female patient with a history of glioma is currently undergoing chemotherapy. The patient was discharged from the hospital to hospice 5 days later when she started having a strange mild cognitive change, suicidal thoughts, and altered mental status. Which of the following options can explain this patient's strange behavior?

    (a) Hypocalcemia
    (b) Steroid psychosis
    (c) Hypernatremia
    (d) Hyperglycemia
    (e) Vincristine encephalitis

    Answer: b

    Hypocalcemia can result from tumor lysis syndrome, a complication of chemotherapy. Other options do not apply here. Therefore, the usage of high doses of steroids such as dexamethasone can cause cognitive changes such as psychosis.

32. A 45-year-old female presents with an ongoing onset of blurry vision and severe headache. The patient is currently undergoing chemotherapy for ovarian cancer. On examination, the patient appears to have bilateral papilledema. Which of the following might help in improving the patient's condition?

    (a) Diuretics
    (b) Carbonic anhydrase inhibitor
    (c) Corticosteroids
    (d) Tetracycline
    (e) None of the above

    Answer: c

    The patient's symptoms mostly describe a common mild visual impairment during chemotherapy known as Carboplatin-Induced Bilateral Papilledema. Although no treatment has been shown to be effective, in certain cases, an empiric corticosteroid is suggested. Similarly, the patient's condition can be confused with idiopathic intracranial hypertension (IIH), which occurs due to a high pressure could be caused by CSF buildup located in the subarachnoid space. It is common among the female gender (20–50 years old). Acetazolamide is an example of a diuretic and carbonic anhydrase inhibitor medication that treats the symptoms caused by IIH.

33. A 57-year-old female patient with persistent glioblastoma has been transferred to hospice care. Her daughter called to state that recently all the mother desires

to do is nap during the day as well as nights of sleep for 13–14 h up to the following day. What should be the next step in the management?

(a) Provide frequent position changes to maintain good skincare
(b) Continue anticonvulsants if the patient can swallow
(c) Continue steroids if the patient can swallow
(d) Position the head of the bed at 30 degrees
(e) All of the above are correct

Answer: e

Drowsiness is one of the main often-reported symptoms that glioblastoma patients experience in their final weeks of life. Great care should be delivered to retain skin integrity as well as prevent aspiration by positioning the head of the bed at 30 degrees. Lastly, if the patient can swallow, anticonvulsants and steroids can be used to improve the patient's symptoms only for a short time.

Test your learning and check your understanding of this book's contents: use the "Springer Nature Flashcards" app to access questions using https://sn.pub/3HwHCw To use the app, please follow the instructions in Chap. 1.

Bibliography

1. Prayson RA. Neuropathology. In: A volume in the series: foundations in diagnostic pathology. 2nd ed. Philadelphia, PA: Elsevier; 2012.
2. Stupp R, Mason WP, van den Bent MJ, et al. Radiotherapy plus concomitant and adjuvant temozolomide for glioblastoma. N Engl J Med. 2005;352:987–96.
3. Pace A, Lorenzo CD, Guariglia L, Jandolo B, Carapella CM, Pompili A. End of life issues in brain tumor patients. J Neuro-Oncol. 2009;91:39–43.
4. Walbert T, Khan M. End-of-life symptoms and care in patients with primary malignant brain tumors: a systematic literature review. J Neuro-Oncol. 2014;117(2):217–24. https://doi.org/10.1007/s11060-014-1393-6.
5. Cohn M, Calton B, Chang S, Page M. Transitions in care for patients with brain tumors: palliative and hospice care. San Francisco, CA: Neuro-Oncology Gordon Murray Caregiver Program, Department of Neurological Surgery, University of California San Francisco; 2014.
6. Abernathy AP, Wheeler JL, Kamal A, Currow DC. When should corticosteroids be used to manage pain? In: Goldstein NE, Morrison RS, editors. Evidence- based practice in palliative medicine. Philadelphia, PA: Elsevier; 2013. p. 44–8.
7. Weller M, Gorlia T, Cairncross JG, van den Bent MJ, Mason W, Belanger K, Brandes AA, Bogdahn U, Macdonald DR, Forsyth P, Rossetti AO, Lacombe D, Mirimanoff RO, Vecht CJ, Stupp R. Prolonged survival with valproic acid use in the EORTC/NCIC temozolomide trial for glioblastoma. Neurology. 2011;77(12):1156–64. https://doi.org/10.1212/WNL.0b013e31822f02e1. Epub 2011 Aug 31. PMID: 21880994; PMCID: PMC3265044.
8. Younus J, Collins A, Wang X, Saunders M, Manuel J, Freake C, Defen P. A double blind placebo controlled pilot study to evaluate the effect of ginseng on fatigue and quality of life in adult chemo-naïve cancer patients. Proc Am Soc Clin Oncol. 2003;22:733.
9. Pace A, Metro G, Fabi A. Supportive care in neurooncology. Curr Opin Oncol. 2010;22:621–6.
10. Newton HB. Supportive care in neuro-oncology. In: Mehta M, editor. Principles and practice of neuro-oncology. New York, NY: Demos Medical; 2014. p. 304–10.

11. Sizoo EM, Braam L, Postma TJ, et al. Symptoms and problems in the end-of-life phase of high-grade glioma patients. Neuro-Oncology. 2010;12(11):1162–6. https://doi.org/10.1093/neuonc/nop045.

12. Ford E, Catt S, Chalmers A, Fallowfield L. Systematic review of supportive care needs in patients with primary malignant brain tumors. Neuro-Oncology. 2012;14:392–404.

13. Witteler J, Schild SE, Rades D. Prognostic factors of local control and survival in patients irradiated for glioblastoma multiforme (GBM). Anticancer Res. 2020;40:7025–30.

14. Galicich J, French LA, Melby JC. Use of dexamethasone in treatment of cerebral edema associated with brain tumors. J Lancet. 1961;81:46–53.

15. Agnelli G, Verso M. Thromboprophylaxis during chemotherapy after advanced cancer. Thromb Res. 2007;120:S128–32.

16. Perry J, Rogers L, Laperriere N, Julian J, Geerts W, Agnelli G, Malkin M, Sawaya R, Baker R, Levine M. PRODIGE: A phase III randomized placebo-controlled trial of thromboprophylaxis using dalteparin low molecular weight heparin (LMWH) in patients with newly diagnosed malignant glioma. J Clin Oncol. 2007;25:2011.

17. Streiff MB, Ye X, Kickler TS, Desideri S, Jani J, Fisher J, Grossman SA. A prospective multicenter study of venous thromboembolism in patients with newly-diagnosed high-grade glioma: hazard rate and risk factors. J Neuro-Oncol. 2015;124:299–305.

18. Youssef J, Novosad SA, Winthrop KL. Infection risk and safety of corticosteroid use. Rheum Dis Clin North Am. 2016;42(1):157–76. https://doi.org/10.1016/j.rdc.2015.08.004. ix–x Epub 2015 Oct 24. PMID: 26611557; PMCID: PMC4751577.

19. Tasaka S. Pneumocystis pneumonia in human immunodeficiency virus-infected adults and adolescents: current concepts and future directions. Clin Med Insights Circ Respir Pulm Med. 2015;9(Suppl 1):19–28. https://doi.org/10.4137/CCRPM.S23324. PMID: 26327786; PMCID: PMC4536784.

20. Hegi ME, Diserens A-C, Gorlia T, Hamou M-F, de Tribolet N, Weller M, Kros JM, Hainfellner JA, Mason W, Mariani L. MGMT gene silencing and benefit from temozolomide in glioblastoma. N Engl J Med. 2005;352:997–1003.

21. Gramatzki D, Roth P, Rushing E, Weller J, Andratschke N, Hofer S, Korol D, Regli L, Pangalu A, Pless M. Bevacizumab may improve quality of life, but not overall survival in glioblastoma: an epidemiological study. Ann Oncol. 2018;29:1431–6.

22. Kaal EC, Vecht CJ. The management of brain edema in brain tumors. Curr Opin Oncol. 2004;16:593–600.

23. Coomans MB, van der Linden SD, Gehring K, Taphoorn MJB. Treatment of cognitive deficits in brain tumour patients: current status and future directions. Curr Opin Oncol. 2019;31(6):540–7. https://doi.org/10.1097/CCO.0000000000000581. PMID: 31483326; PMCID: PMC6824580.

24. Fischer N, Stuermer J, Rodic B, Pless M. Carboplatin-induced bilateral papilledema: a case report. Case Rep Oncol. 2009;2(1):67–71. https://doi.org/10.1159/000212087. PMID: 20740148; PMCID: PMC2918832

25. Mollan SP, Davies B, Silver NC, Shaw S, Mallucci CL, Wakerley BR, Krishnan A, Chavda SV, Ramalingam S, Edwards J, Hemmings K, Williamson M, Burdon MA, Hassan-Smith G, Digre K, Liu GT, Jensen RH, Sinclair AJ. Idiopathic intracranial hypertension: consensus guidelines on management. J Neurol Neurosurg Psychiatry. 2018;89(10):1088–100. https://doi.org/10.1136/jnnp-2017-317440. Epub 2018 Jun 14. PMID: 29903905; PMCID: PMC6166610.

Printed in the United States
by Baker & Taylor Publisher Services